Perspectives in
Trypanosomiasis
Research

TROPICAL MEDICINE RESEARCH STUDIES SERIES

Series Editor: **Dr. K. N. Brown**
National Institute for Medical Research, England

1. Schistosoma Mansoni: The Parasite Surface in Relation to Host Immunity
    Diane J. McLaren

2. The Biology of *Entamoeba histolytica*
    Adolfo Martinez-Palomo

3. Perspectives in Trypanosomiasis Research
    Edited by **John R. Baker**

Perspectives in Trypanosomiasis Research

PROCEEDINGS OF THE TWENTY-FIRST
TRYPANOSOMIASIS SEMINAR: LONDON,
24 SEPTEMBER, 1981

Edited by
John R. Baker, D.Sc.
Culture Centre of Algae and Protozoa,
Institute of Terrestrial Ecology,
Natural Environment Research Council,
Cambridge, England

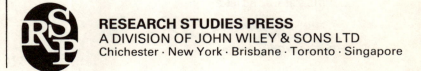

RESEARCH STUDIES PRESS
A DIVISION OF JOHN WILEY & SONS LTD
Chichester · New York · Brisbane · Toronto · Singapore

RESEARCH STUDIES PRESS

Editorial Office:
58B Station Road, Letchworth, Herts. SG6 3BE, England

British Library Cataloguing in Publication Data:

Trypanosomiasis Seminar *(21st: 1981; London)*
Perspectives in trypanosomiasis research.—
(Tropical medicine research studies series; 3)
1. Trypanosomiasis—Congresses
I. Title   II. Baker, John R.   III. Series
616.9'363   RC186.3

ISBN 0 471 10478 7 /

Printed in Great Britain

Preface

The first of what was to become an annual series of seminars on trypanosomiasis was held at the National Institute for Medical Research in London, on 27 October 1970, under the auspices of the (then) Colonial Office of the British Government. Its published proceedings, though brief, by now constitute a document of some historical interest - even though it gives me a wrong second initial (see bibliography). Seminars were held annually thereafter, organized by the Colonial Office and its successors, the Ministry of Overseas Development and the Overseas Development Administration (ODA) of the Foreign and Commonwealth Office, until 1979, when the venue was Bristol. Plans were well under way for the 1980 meeting when the worsening financial crisis in Britain forced the ODA to withdraw its support, and no meeting was held. However, the cessation of what had become a respected and internationally attended event was regretted by many, and thanks to the initiative and enthusiasm of the officers of the British Society for Parasitology and the Royal Society of Tropical Medicine and Hygiene, the generosity of the latter society in providing accommodation at Manson House in London, and the industry of Dr D.G. Godfrey in arranging the programme, the twenty-first seminar was held on 24 September 1981.

The general theme of the meeting was current inadequacies in trypanosomiasis and tsetse research and control. The organisers' intention was to emphasize fields of research which, while of proven worth, were perhaps in danger of being neglected in the present wave of (entirely justified) enthusiasm for more 'fashionable' topics such as molecular biology. Three sessions were held, consisting of short papers by invited contributors on trypanosomiasis, chemotherapy, and tsetse, under the chairmanship of, respectively, myself, Dr J. Williamson and Dr A.M. Jordan. Following these talks, an evening poster session took place at the London School of Hygiene and Tropical Medicine. The meeting was attended by some 150 people, and was generally judged a great success. Originally no plan was made for the publication of the proceedings, but there was a general demand for this and, thanks to the efforts of Dr K.N. Brown and Research Studies Press, the demand has been met. This book is the result: it contains the substance of the talks by the invited speakers - to whom thanks are due for their promptness in producing written versions of their contributions so unexpectedly and hurriedly. Thanks are also due to Mrs G. Coulson for her speedy and accurate typing.

In conclusion, I wish to join with the many attenders at the seminar in expressing a fervent wish for the continuation of this annual event - resurrected significantly perhaps at its 'coming of age' - by private enterprise, if not by governmental support.

J.R. Baker

Bibliography

The first seminar was reported in the Annals of Tropical Medicine and Parasitology. After that, publication apparently lapsed but was recommenced with seminar no. 6 in the Transactions of the Royal Society of Tropical Medicine and Hygiene. References to these reports are given below.

Annals of Tropical Medicine and Parasitology, 1961, 55, 133-150

Transactions of the Royal Society of Tropical Medicine and Hygiene,

1966, 60, 117-127;	1967, 61, 131-147;	1968, 62, 120-147;
1969, 63, 112-130;	1970, 64, 159-188;	1971, 65, 214-266;
1972, 66, 324-355;	1973, 67, 254-306;	1974, 68, 145-163;
1975, 69, 266-284;	1976, 70, 114-129;	1977, 71, 1-15;
1978, 72, 109-122;	1979, 73, 125-139;	1980, 74, 267-282.

Table of Contents

CHAPTER 1
Trypanosoma cruzi:
Epidemiology

Michael A. Miles

Department of Medical Protozoology,
London School of Hygiene and Tropical Medicine,
Keppel Street, London, WC1E 7HT.

1.1. Introduction

Trypanosoma cruzi, the aetiological agent of Chagas's disease, is widely distributed in the Americas. Infections are known from well over one hundred mammal species of eight orders (Hoare 1972; Barretto and Ribeiro 1979). Human infection is endemic throughout major regions of South and Central America but, despite the abundance of silvatic transmission, is only sporadic in North America (Miles 1979). Imported cases, such as those seen recently in Canada (Schipper *et al*. 1980) are becoming more frequent as immigration and leisure travel increases.

T. cruzi is not transmitted directly by the bite of infected triatomine vectors (Hemiptera, Reduviidae) but by contamination of mucous membranes or abraded skin with infected bug faeces. Infective (metacyclic) trypanosomes often penetrate the conjunctiva or the wound of the triatomine bite. Bug faeces are irritant, which aids dispersion to these sites; many vector species defaecate during or just after feeding. Trypomastigotes invade reticulo-endothelial cells locally, multiply and may produce lesions such as unilateral conjunctivitis, (Romaña's sign) if the site of infection is the eye, or a cutaneous 'chagoma'. The early or acute phase of infection may vary in severity from being quite inapparent to fatal and may include symptoms such as fever, lymphadenopathy, malaise and ECG abnormalities. Subsequent phases of infection are the indeterminate phase, without symptoms, which may last for many years or be life-long, and the chronic phase, which may feature ECG abnormalities, megacardia, aperistalsis, megaoesophagus and megacolon. Direct transmission from man to man may occur by transfusion of infected blood; there is also a small amount of congenital transmission.

There are about a hundred species of triatomine vector worldwide

(Miles 1979; Lent and Wygodzinsky 1979); most are confined to the
Americas and the majority of these have been found naturally infected
with *T. cruzi*. The six principal vectors of human disease, those
that readily colonize houses and feed from man and his domestic
animals, are: *Triatoma infestans* in Argentina, Bolivia, Brazil, Chile,
Paraguay, Peru and Uruguay; *Panstrongylus megistus* in central and
eastern Brazil; *T. brasiliensis* in northeastern Brazil; *T. sordida*,
often sympatric with *T. infestans*; *Rhodnius prolixus* in Colombia,
Ecuador, Venezuela and parts of Central America; and *T. dimidiata* in
Central and the extreme north of South America. The natural habitats,
or presumed natural habitats, of these vectors are often reflected in
the type of household infestation. Thus domestic *R. prolixus* predom-
inates in palm roofs and palm trees are its natural ecotope. Domestic
and silvatic transmission cycles may be entirely separate or linked
by the replenishment of household vector colonies from silvatic foci
(Miles 1979).

Understanding of the regional epidemiology of Chagas's disease is
largely a function of the extent of local investigations. Epidemiological studies have been undertaken for many years in Brazil,
Venezuela and large parts of Argentina and Chile (Figure 1) (Haddock
1979). Elsewhere national effort has been, often understandably, less
intense, although there are several examples of excellent research
projects or valiant control programmes in high risk zones (Gonzalez
1978; Goldsmith *et al*. 1978; Muynck 1977). It is possible to obtain
a good picture of the prevalence of human infection in several countries of South America. If sufficient information is available, this
is best done from a systematic nationwide serological survey, such as
that undertaken in Brazil (Castro and Silveira 1979). Alternatively
one or two serological samples, together with a knowledge of vector
and human population distribution, can give a reasonable idea of
prevalence. Figure 2 presents estimates for several South American
countries, but three with extensive endemic areas (Ecuador, Peru and
Uruguay) are excluded due to insufficient data. Whilst prevalence
estimates for each country do vary widely (for example down to 0.56
million for Venezuela and up to 2.3 million for Argentina) it is
apparent that approximately 10 million individuals on the South American
continent must carry *T. cruzi* (Urribarri and Soto 1976; Schenone *et
al*. 1978; D'Alessandro *et al*. 1971; Castro and Silveira 1979; Miles
1979).

1.2. Epidemiological gaps

Clearly there are many inadequacies in our knowledge and understanding
of all the intricacies of *T. cruzi* epidemiology. It seems to me, from
several years of Chagas's disease research, and from reading many
relevant publications, that there are three large areas in which additional information would be welcomed as enhancing prospects for control, of both individual cases and endemic disease.

The lack of information on the significance of Chagas's disease as
a public health problem in the less well studied areas of South

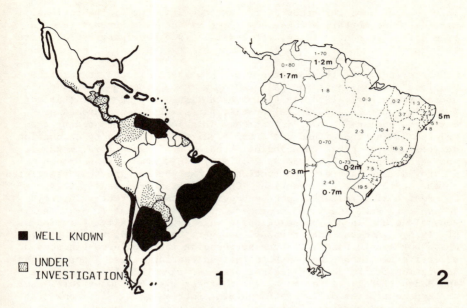

Figure 1.   The distribution of Chagas's disease research.   Detailed
   studies have continued in Brazil, Venezuela, Argentina and Chile
   for many years;   other areas are less well studied (modified from
   Haddock 1979).

Figure 2.   The estimated prevalence of human *T. cruzi* infection in
   South America.   Estimates for each country vary substantially (for
   example, down to 0.56 million in Venezuela and up to 2.3 million in
   Argentina).   Absence of an entry does not necessarily imply absence
   of the infection.   A total of about 10 million individuals on the
   South American continent carry *T. cruzi*.   (Totals are in millions;
   smaller numbers indicate seropositivity rates for Brazil or, for
   other countries, range of seropositivity rates.   Based on literature
   cited in the text.)

America requires action. The first step in this direction is to
establish the prevalence of infection (not necessarily of disease) by
screening an appropriate collection of finger-prick or venous blood
samples for the presence of *T. cruzi* antibody; several reliable
serological methods are available (Miles 1979). In this context Brazil,
the largest and one of the richer countries of South America, has
pointed the way by screening blood samples from every state. In conjunction with the collection of blood samples, selected households can
be surveyed easily for the presence of vectors. Public health organizations are sufficiently well organized throughout much of South
America, as the aftermath of malaria or arbovirus control programmes,
to cope with this service. This is a relatively simple and straight-

forward approach, far removed from an understanding of the regional
morbidity and mortality caused by *T. cruzi* and even further removed
from effective control. Nevertheless, it is a necessary prerequisite
to both these goals.

Understanding of the pathogenesis of Chagas's disease is far from
complete. The elegant and painstaking work of Köberle and his collaborators (Köberle 1968, 1974) has established beyond doubt that, at
least in southern and central Brazil, parasympathetic neurones are
destroyed during *T. cruzi* infection. This loss, exacerbated by age-
related diminution of neurones, can be directly related to conduction
defects and the gross pathological syndromes of megacardia, megacolon
and megaoesophagus (Andrade *et al.* 1978). How are these neurones
destroyed, and is their destruction, as has been suggested, restricted
to the acute phase of infection? One mechanism proposed is that a
T. cruzi toxin, released upon pseudocyst rupture, directly destroys
adjacent tissue, including neurones. It is clear that *T. cruzi* antigens alone can induce pathological change experimentally (Teixeira *et
al.* 1975). A different proposal, however, is that adsorption of *T.
cruzi* antigen to normal tissues surrounding infected areas induces a
selective autoimmune response to antigen bearing cells; such antigen
adsorption can be readily demonstrated *in vitro* (Ribeiro dos Santos
and Hudson 1980). A yet more radical theory is that amastigotes and/
or trypomastigotes of *T. cruzi* contain, intrinsically, antigens that
cross-react with normal host components and induce a chronic autoimmune disease. Teixeira *et al.* (1975) and Teixeira (1979) explored
this concept in depth and found destruction *in vitro* of normal heart
cells by *T. cruzi*-sensitized lymphocytes from experimentally infected
rabbits. Two of these mechanisms of pathogenesis, neurone destruction
by an endotoxin and antigen adsorption, imply that most damage is done
in the acute phase of infection, whilst the concept of Chagas's disease as a chronic autoimmune process suggests a continuous pathogenesis.
Post mortem evidence can be found to support pathogenesis in the acute
phase and a progressive pathogenesis (Miles 1979). Hudson (1981), in
a pertinent review, concluded from experimental studies in mice that
neurone destruction occurs in the late acute phase during the resol-
ution of parasitaemia, and that cell mediated autoimmunity emerges
after neurone destruction. Both post mortem and clinical methods of
assessment have improved radically over the last few years due to
technical, analytical and theoretical innovation. This progress is
now being exploited, for example in studies of neurotransmitter
depletion in Chagas's disease (Long *et al.* 1980). In parallel with
such investigations of the pathogenesis of Chagas's disease there is
a need for further development of a satisfactory animal model of the
chronic phase (Miles *et al.* 1979).

Directly relevant to the pathogenesis of Chagas's disease is the
enduring enigma of regional differences in the chronic pathology.
'Mega' syndromes are commonly seen in central and southern Brazil;
records of hundreds of individual cases are found in the literature
and corrective surgical procedures are highly developed (Rassi 1979).
In contrast, mega syndromes do not appear to be a feature of Chagas's

disease in Venezuela despite the examination of many thousands of cases (Rezende 1976; Miles 1979). Cerisola *et al*. (1977) have, by similar comparative studies of chemotherapy in Argentina, Chile and Brazil, confirmed disparities in cure rates with nifurtimox. Other circumstantial evidence of *T. cruzi* heterogeneity has been reviewed recently (Miles 1979).

This appraisal of three main epidemiological gaps, namely: lack of full appreciation of (a) distribution and prevalence, (b) the mechanisms of pathogenesis of chronic disease and (c) the geograph-ical variations in clinical form, is in alignment with priorities assigned by the World Health Organization (1980). The last two of these gaps are closely linked. Comparative pathological and clinical re-evaluation of Chagas's disease in selected regions such as Venezuela, central and southern Brazil and a third area in the Andean region, with international participants, would be a valuable approach. With various collaborators I have been involved in the biochemical assess-ment of *T. cruzi* heterogeneity, to determine whether strain differences may possibly explain regional differences in Chagas's disease, and should be considered in other aspects of host-parasite relationship and the development of measures towards control.

1.3. *T. cruzi* zymodemes

Enzyme electrophoresis has changed specific and sub-specific tax-onomy of many parasitic protozoa. The major relationships indicated by biochemical characters have, however, more often than not confirmed classical or intuitive groupings. The enzyme profiles of more than three hundred newly isolated *T. cruzi* stocks have been determined with up to 18 enzymes. The *T. cruzi* stocks were isolated, not only from areas with separate, overlapping or enzootic transmission cycles, but from two regions, Venezuela and parts of Brazil, with allegedly very different forms of chronic Chagas's disease. The results of these studies have been described in detail (Miles *et al*. 1980a, 1981a, 1981b) and will not be repeated here. The main conclusions from these investigations were the usefulness of stable enzyme characters in identifying strains and unravelling local epidemiologies, and the identification of at least 3 major, radically dissimilar zymodemes, in central and northern Brazil and Venezuela. These zymodemes, named Z1, Z2 and Z3, had very different geographical distributions (Figure 3, Table 1). Endemic Chagas's disease in Venezuela was mainly due to Z1 whereas Z2, not found in Venezuela, was isolated from many patients in eastern and central Brazil. There was some indication that Z1 and Z3 were associated with different silvatic mammals in enzootic trans-mission in the Brazilian Amazon basin. The observed distribution of *T. cruzi* zymodemes supported the idea of separate and overlapping domestic and silvatic transmission cycles, confirmed the origins of sporadic cases in the Amazon basin and, above all, provided circum-stantial evidence that regional differences in the manifestation of *T. cruzi* infection might be strain-dependent (Table 1).

A simplistic view of the *T. cruzi* zymodemes would be to assume that

	MAN	DOMESTIC	SILVATIC
VENEZUELA	Z1: 18 Z3: 1	Z1: 13	Z1: 19 Z3: 1
BRAZIL - Amazon basin	Z1: 3 Z3: 4	NOT PRESENT	Z1: 106 Z3: 12 Z3/Z1 ASAT: 6
BRAZIL - central and eastern	Z1: 1 Z2: 98	Z2: 9	Z1: 23 Z3: 2

Table 1. Major zymodeme categories of 316 stocks of *T. cruzi* from
   Venezuela and Brazil. (Slightly modified, by permission, from
   Lancet, 20 June 1981.)

they were distinct taxa. The degree of difference between enzyme
profiles of South American species or subspecies of *Leishmania* are
similar to the degree of difference between *T. cruzi* zymodemes.
Leishmania mexicana amazonensis is separated from *L. hertigi* by
eleven enzymes and from *L. braziliensis* by ten of fourteen enzymes;
L. b. braziliensis is separated from *L. b. guyanensis* by four of
fourteen enzymes; *L. h. hertigi* is separated from *L. h. deanei* by
three of eighteen (Miles *et al*. 1980b, 1981c). The corresponding
differences for *T. cruzi* zymodemes are: Z1 from Z2, ten of eighteen
enzymes; Z2 from Z3, nine of eighteen enzymes; and Z1 from Z3 eight
of eighteen enzymes (Miles *et al*. 1980a). A simple numerical taxonomic approach confirmed the radical differences between the *T. cruzi*
zymodemes (Ready and Miles 1980). The *Leishmania* taxa can be separated
from each other by several behavioural and epidemiological characters
as well as enzyme profiles (Miles *et al*. 1981c). Such defined biological parameters are not available for *T. cruzi* strains, although
one, doubling time, has emerged from growth studies *in vitro* of zymodeme clones (Dvorak *et al*. 1980).

What is the relationship between the *T. cruzi* zymodemes, are we to
consider them as unnamed taxa? This is the obvious conclusion from
present limited observations but may be short-sighted. Figure 4 shows
the patterns of two enzymes, PGM and GPI, for Z1 and Z2. In man,
PGM is a monomer and GPI a dimer. If we assume that these enzymes
have the same subunit structure in *T. cruzi* as in man, Z1 and Z2 may
be homozygotes related to each other through undescribed heterozygotes
(Figure 4, centre). Putative homozygous and heterozygous forms of a
tetrameric enzyme are also shown in Figure 4. Heterozygous patterns
are derived from different alleles at a single locus in a diploid
organism but may result from different loci in a haploid organism.
Typical heterozygous GPI patterns have emerged during recent studies
of *T. cruzi* stocks from Bolivia (Tibayrenc *et al*. 1981). Clearly

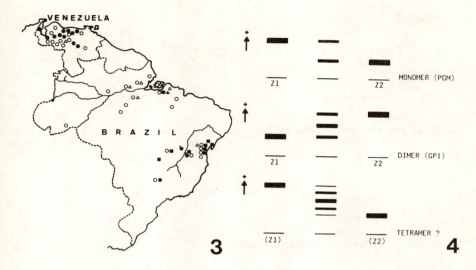

Figure 3.   Distribution of three *T. cruzi* zymodemes (Z1-Z3) in Venezuela and Brazil.   ●Z1 in man;   ■Z2 in man;   ▲Z3 in man;   ○Z1
silvatic and   △Z3 silvatic.   (Reproduced by permission from Lancet,
20 June 1981.)

Figure 4.   Diagram of profiles produced by starch-gel electrophoresis
of 2 enzymes (phosphoglucomutase, PGM and glucose phosphate isomerase, GPI) from 2 zymodemes of *T. cruzi* (Z1 and Z2).   Hypothetical
heterozygous patterns are shown between the observed (homozygous?)
profiles;   putative homozygous and heterozygous patterns for a
postulated tetrameric enzyme are also shown.

then our interpretation of *T. cruzi* zymodemes and understanding of
T. cruzi epidemiology is severely hindered by the absence of fundamental
information on the nature of the *T. cruzi* genome and modes of reproduction.

1.4.   The relevance of fundamental studies

  There is a natural tendency to think of the protozoa as being both
small and simple.   In fact their diversity and complexity are aston-
ishing.   They show great divergence in DNA organization with remarkable
variation in the mechanics and orchestration of sexual reproduction.
Some of the range of protozoan attributes are summarized in Figure 5.
It is not clear which of these attributes are to be assigned to *T. cruzi*;
the organism has been considered to be haploid and asexual (Sleigh
1979), but this is questionable.   Several approaches can be exploited
to clarify the basic biology of *T. cruzi* and gain insight into its
epidemiology, particularly the question of infraspecific variation.

8

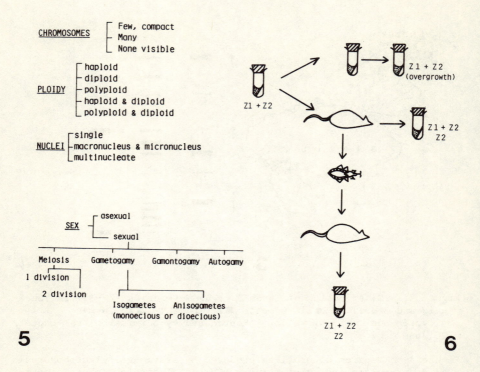

CHROMOSOMES — Few, compact
— Many
— None visible

PLOIDY — haploid
— diploid
— polyploid
— haploid & diploid
— polyploid & diploid

NUCLEI — single
— macronucleus & micronucleus
— multinucleate

SEX — asexual
— sexual

Meiosis   Gametogamy   Gamontogamy   Autogamy
1 division
2 division
Isogametes   Anisogametes
(monoecious or dioecious)

Z1 + Z2

Z1 + Z2
(overgrowth)

Z1 + Z2
Z2

Z1 + Z2
Z2

5   6

Figure 5.   A summary of the diversity of genomes and modes of reproduction found within the protozoa (from data by Sleigh 1979).

Figure 6.   Design of one mixed zymodeme transmission experiment to
investigate possibility of recombination between *T. cruzi* zymodemes.
In the experiment shown, *T. cruzi* Z1 and Z2 were passaged from
culture to mouse to bug to mouse and back into culture; no new
enzyme band was found.

One or two examples only, using enzymes and DNA analyses, are given to
illustrate this point.

The natural distribution of enzyme profiles, the presence of heterozygous patterns and Hardy-Weinberg equilibria can help to establish
relationships between zymodemes (Tait 1980; Godfrey, this volume,
chapter 4). Enzymes can also be used experimentally as markers in
attempts to generate recombinant forms between zymodemes. Accordingly,
we have recently performed a series of transmission experiments using
zymodeme mixtures; part of one of these is shown in Figure 6. Bi-
phasic agar cultures of *T. cruzi* Z1 and Z2, past their exponential
growth period and containing trypomastigotes, were mixed and passaged
from mouse to triatomine bug, to mouse again and back into cultures.

Mixtures were also re-isolated by culture from the first mouse passage or maintained in culture together for long periods. Overgrowth, attributable to shorter Z1 doubling times (Dvorak *et al.* 1980) was observed in mixed cultures. No new enzyme band to suggest recombination could be found in concentrated enzyme extracts after transmission *in vivo* or maintenance *in vitro*.

Analysis of enzyme subunit structures can be used to question the validity of genetic interpretations of presumed heterozygous patterns in *T. cruzi*. The production of such patterns depends on multimeric enzymes. An indication of subunit structures can be obtained from comparative estimates of enzyme molecular size in man and *T. cruzi*. In a recent preliminary study Jeremiah *et al.* (in press) found that molecular weight estimates of seven of eight enzymes were of the same order of magnitude as their human equivalents, implying a similar subunit structure.

DNA analyses are perhaps the ultimate approach to a detailed understanding of the *T. cruzi* genome. Dvorak and his colleagues at the National Institutes of Health, Bethesda, have begun to use the fluorescent activated cell sorter (FACS) in quantitating the DNA of *T. cruzi* zymodeme clones, revealing interesting relationships (Dvorak, J.A., personal communication). This extraordinary machine has the capacity not only to analyse, but also to sort, extremely rapidly, single cells on the basis of light scatter and fluorescence. The potential application in the study of parasitic protozoa are enormous. Lanar *et al.* (1981) have used DNA reassociation studies and microspectrofluorometric quantitation of DNA to probe the *T. cruzi* genome. In support of evidence from putative heterozygous bands and enzyme molecular size estimates they too conclude that *T. cruzi* is 'most likely a diploid organism'.

Solari (1980) has sought direct evidence of the chromatin constitution of *T. cruzi* by the three dimensional reconstitution of mitotic nuclei from serial sections. Chromatin remains dispersed throughout nuclear division but ten equatorial dense plaques were observed. These plaques split at the beginning of elongation and migrate to the nuclear poles, suggesting a kinetochore-like function, and therefore, the existence of ten chromosome units.

1.5. Definition of strains

Definition of infraspecific variation in *T. cruzi* was, for many years, unsuccessful due to the lack of stable intrinsic parameters. The position is now quite the reverse. This problem can be approached now with a whole battery of procedures such as enzyme electrophoresis, which can be performed in field situations (Lanham *et al.* 1981); quantitation and analysis of DNA, both kinetoplastic and nuclear, for example using restriction endonucleases (Borst *et al.* 1980; Morel *et al.* 1980); SDS-PAGE peptide profiling (Araujo and Remington, 1981); lectin analyses of carbohydrate receptors (Pereira *et al.* 1980); and, most significant of all, monoclonal antibodies. The latter promise

10

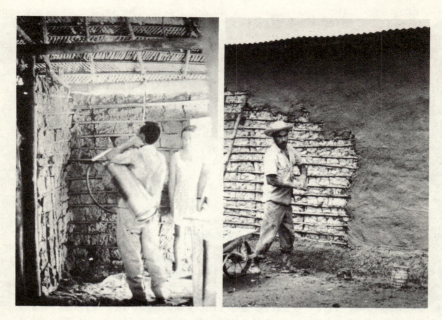

Figure 7. Insecticide application (left) and surveillance and self
help housing improvement (right), proven practical methods of control
of *T. cruzi* infection not always adequately employed (see text).

not only simple identification of taxa and strains but have the most
profound importance in directing the search for potent, harmless
immunogens (Miles in press).

1.6. The principal 'epidemiological inadequacy'

It has been established that endemic Chagas's disease can be controlled by a combination of judicious application of selected insecticides, surveillance and self-reliant housing improvement (Figure 7).
Dias (1978) has produced detailed guidelines for such means of control,
made cost-effective by involvement of local inhabitants. On a larger
scale the control of endemic Chagas's disease in São Paulo State has
been extremely successful. The most appropriate means of control are
indeed well known (Miles *et al.* 1981d). In the same way, infected
donor blood, which may be used in 7-10% of transfusions in some areas
(Baruffa 1979; Apt *et al.* 1980), can be made safe effectively, if not
ideally (Cruz *et al.* 1980; Gutteridge, Chapter 5, this volume). There
is no question that the most striking 'epidemiological inadequacy' is
the failure to use these proven methods of control to limit the spread
of Chagas's disease.

Acknowledgements

I thank the Lancet for permission to reproduce Figure 3 and Table 1.
I am extremely grateful to the Wellcome Trust for their financial
support.

1.7. References

Andrade, Z.A., Andrade, S.G., Oliveira, G.B. and Alonso, D.R. (1978).
  Histopathology of the conducting tissue of the heart in Chagas'
  myocarditis. American Heart Journal 95, 316-324.

Apt, W., Perez, C. and Sandoval, J. (1980). Prevalence of Chagas'
  infection in four blood banks of different geographic areas in Chile.
  Revista Medica de Chile 108, 112-114.

Araujo, F.G. and Remington, J.S. (1981). Characterization of stages
  and strains of *Trypanosoma cruzi* by analysis of cell membrane
  components. Journal of Immunology 127, 855-859.

Barretto, M.P. and Ribeiro, R.D. (1979). Reservatórios silvestres
  do *Trypanosoma (Schizotrypanum) cruzi* Chagas, 1909. Revista do
  Instituto Adolfo Lutz 39, 25-36.

Baruffa, G. (1979). Prevalência da infecção chagásica no banco de
  sangue da Santa Casa de Misericórdia de Pelotas, Rio Grande do Sul,
  Brasil. Revista do Instituto de Medicina Tropical de São Paulo 21,
  37-42.

Borst, P., Fase-Fowler, A., Frasch, A.C.C., Hoeijmakers, J.H.J. and
  Weijers, P.J. (1980). Characterization of DNA from *Trypanosoma
  brucei* and related trypanosomes by restriction endonuclease digestion.
  Molecular and Biochemical Parasitology 1, 221-246.

Castro Filho, J. de and Silveira, A.C. (1979). Distribuição da doença
  de Chagas no Brasil. Revista Brasileira de Malariologia e Doenças
  Tropicais 31, 85-97.

Cerisola, J.A., Neves da Silva, N., Prata, A., Schenone, H. and
  Rohwedder, R. (1977). Evaluation of the efficacy of nifurtimox
  in chronic human chagasic infection by using xenodiagnosis.
  Boletin Chileno de Parasitologia 32, 51-62.

Cruz, F.S., Marr, J.J. and Berens, R.L. (1980). Prevention of transfusion-induced Chagas' disease by amphotericin B. American Journal
  of Tropical Medicine and Hygiene 29, 761-765.

D'Alessandro, A., Barretto, P. and Duarte, C.A. (1971). Distribution
  of triatomine-transmitted trypanosomiasis in Colombia and new
  records of the bugs and infections. Journal of Medical Entomology
  8, 159-172.

Dias, J.C.P. and Garcia, A.L.R. (1978). Vigilancia epidemiologica
  con participacion comunitaria. Un programa de enfermedad de Chagas.
  Boletin de la Oficina Sanitaria Panamericana 84, 533-544.

Dvorak, J.A., Hartmann, D.L. and Miles, M.A. (1980). *Trypanosoma cruzi*: correlation of growth kinetics to zymodeme type in clones derived from various sources. Journal of Protozoology 27, 472-474.

Goldsmith, R.S., Kagan, I.G., Zarate, R., Reyes-Gonzalez, M.A. and Cedeno-Ferreira, J. (1978). Epidemiologic studies of Chagas' disease in Oaxaca, Mexico. Bulletin of the Pan American Health Organization 12, 236-250.

Gonzalez, M.F. (1978). Control de triatomineos con hexaclorociclo-hexano en tres departementos del sur de Peru. Boletin de la Oficina Sanitaria Panamericana 84, 324-331.

Haddock, K.C. (1979). Disease and development in the tropics - a review of Chagas' disease. Social Science and Medicine 13D, 53-60.

Hoare, C.A. (1972). The Trypanosomes of Mammals. Blackwell, Oxford.

Hudson, L. (1981). Immunobiology of *Trypanosoma cruzi* infection and Chagas' disease. Transactions of the Royal Society of Tropical Medicine and Hygiene 75, 493-498.

Jeremiah, S.J., Povey, S. and Miles, M.A. (in press). Support for a genetic interpretation of trypanosome isozymes from a study of molecular size of enzymes in *Trypanosoma cruzi*. Molecular and Biochemical Parasitology.

Köberle, F. (1968). Chagas' disease and Chagas' syndromes: the pathology of American trypanosomiasis. Advances in Parasitology 6, 63-110.

Köberle, F. (1974). Pathogenesis of Chagas' disease, in Trypanosomiasis and Leishmaniasis with special reference to Chagas' disease. (edited by K. Elliott, M. O'Connor and G.E.W. Wolstenholme), Ciba Foundation Symposium 20, pp. 137-158. Associated Scientific Publishers, Amsterdam, London, New York.

Lanar, D.E., Levy, L.S. and Manning, J.E. (1981). Complexity and content of the DNA and RNA in *Trypanosoma cruzi*. Molecular and Biochemical Parasitology 3, 327-341.

Lanham, S.M., Grendon, J.M., Miles, M.A., Póvoa, M.M. and Almeida de Souza, A.A. (1981). A comparison of electrophoretic methods for isoenzyme characterization of trypanosomatids I. Standard stocks of *Trypanosoma cruzi* zymodemes from northeast Brazil. Transactions of the Royal Society of Tropical Medicine and Hygiene 75, 742-750.

Lent, H. and Wygodzinsky, P. (1979). Revision of the Triatominae (Hemiptera, Reduviidae), and their significance as vectors of Chagas' disease. Bulletin of the American Museum of Natural History 163, 1-520.

Long, R.G., Bishop, A.E., Barnes, A.J., Albuquerque, R.H., O'Shaughnessy, D.J., McGregor, G.P., Bannister, R., Polak, J.M. and Bloom, S.R. (1980). Neural and hormonal peptides in rectal biopsy specimens from patients with Chagas' disease and chronic autonomic failure. Lancet, March 15, 559-562.

Miles, M.A. (1979). Transmission cycles and the heterogeneity of *Trypanosoma cruzi*, in Biology of the Kinetoplastida (edited by W.H.R. Lumsden and D.A. Evans), vol. 2, pp. 117-196. Academic Press, London, New York, San Francisco.

Miles, M.A. (in press). The epidemiology of South American trypanosomiasis - biochemical and immunological concepts and their relevance to control. Transactions of the Royal Society of Tropical Medicine and Hygiene.

Miles, M.A., Marsden, P.D., Pettitt, L.E., Draper, C.C., Watson, S., Seah, S.K.K., Hutt, M.S.R. and Fowler, J.M. (1979). Experimental *Trypanosoma cruzi* infection in rhesus monkeys. III. Electrocardiographic and histopathological findings. Transactions of the Royal Society of Tropical Medicine and Hygiene 73, 528-532.

Miles, M.A., Lanham, S.M., Souza, A.A. de, and Póvoa, M. (1980a). Further enzymic characters of *Trypanosoma cruzi* and their evaluation for strain identification. Transactions of the Royal Society of Tropical Medicine and Hygiene 74, 221-237.

Miles, M.A., Póvoa, M.M., Souza, A.A. de, Lainson, R. and Shaw, J.J. (1980b). Some methods for the enzymic characterization of Latin-American *Leishmania* with particular reference to *Leishmania mexicana amazonensis* and subspecies of *Leishmania hertigi*. Transactions of the Royal Society of Tropical Medicine and Hygiene 74, 243-252.

Miles, M.A., Cedillos, R.A., Póvoa, M.M., Souza, A.A. de, Prata, A. and Macedo, V. (1981a). Do radically dissimilar *Trypanosoma cruzi* strains (zymodemes) cause Venezuelan and Brazilian forms of Chagas' disease? Lancet, June 20, 1338-1340.

Miles, M.A., Póvoa, M.M., Souza, A.A. de, Lainson, R., Shaw, J.J. and Ketteridge, D.S. (1981b). Chagas' disease in the Amazon Basin: II. The distribution of *Trypanosoma cruzi* zymodemes 1 and 3 in Pará State, north Brazil. Transactions of the Royal Society of Tropical Medicine and Hygiene 75, 667-674.

Miles, M.A., Lainson, R., Shaw, J.J., Póvoa, M. and Souza, A.A. de (1981c). Leishmaniasis in Brazil: XV. Biochemical distinction of *Leishmania mexicana amazonensis*, *L. braziliensis braziliensis* and *L. braziliensis guyanensis* - aetiological agents of cutaneous leishmaniasis in the Amazon Basin of Brazil. Transactions of the Royal Society of Tropical Medicine and Hygiene 75, 524-529.

Miles, M.A., Souza, A.A. de, and Póvoa, M. (1981d). Chagas' disease in the Amazon Basin. III. Ecotopes of ten triatomine bug species (Hemiptera: Reduviidae) from the vicinity of Belém, Pará State, Brazil. Journal of Medical Entomology 18, 266-278.

Morel, C., Chiari, E., Camargo, E.P., Mattei, D.M., Romanha, A.J. and Simpson, L. (1980). Strains and clones of *Trypanosoma cruzi* can be characterized by pattern of restriction endonuclease products of kinetoplast DNA minicircles. Proceedings of the National Academy of Science, U.S.A. 77, 6810-6814.

Muynck, A. de (1977). Estado actual de conocimientos sobre la problematica de la enfermedad de Chagas en el departamento de Santa Cruz. Boletin Informativo del Cenetrop 3, 41-51.

Pereira, M.E.A., Loures, M.A., Villalta, F. and Andrade, A.F.B. (1980). Lectin receptors as markers for *Trypanosoma cruzi*. Journal of Experimental Medicine 152, 1375-1392.

Rassi, L. (1979). Criterio seletivo na indicacao da tecnica cirurgica para o megaesofago chagasico. Revista Goiania de Medicina 25, 85-104.

Ready, P.D. and Miles, M.A. (1980). Delimitation of *Trypanosoma cruzi* zymodemes by numerical taxonomy. Transactions of the Royal Society of Tropical Medicine and Hygiene 74, 238-242.

Rezende, J.F.M. de (1976). Chagasic mega syndromes and regional differences, in New Approaches in American Trypanosomiasis Research (edited by L.S. Lisann), PAHO Scientific Publication No. 318, pp. 195-205. Pan American Health Organization, Washington.

Ribeiro dos Santos, R. and Hudson, L. (1980). *Trypanosoma cruzi*: immunological consequences of parasite modification of host cells. Clinical and Experimental Immunology 40, 36-41.

Schenone, H., Villarroel, F. and Alfaro, E. (1978). Epidemiología de la enfermedad de Chagas en Chile. Condiciones de la vivienda relacionadas con la presencia de *Triatoma infestans* y la proporción de humanos y animales infectados con *Trypanosoma cruzi*. Boletin Chileno de Parasitologia 33, 2-7.

Schipper, H., McClarty, B.M., McRuer, K.E., Nash, R.A. and Penney, C.H. (1980). Tropical diseases encountered in Canada: 1. Chagas' disease. Canadian Medical Association Journal 122, 165-172.

Sleigh, M. (1979). The Biology of Protozoa. Edward Arnold, London.

Solari, A.J. (1980). The 3-dimensional fine structure of the mitotic spindle in *Trypanosoma cruzi*. Chromosoma 78, 239-255.

Tait, A. (1980). Evidence for diploidy and mating in trypanosomes. Nature 287, 536-538.

Teixeira, A.R.L. (1979). Chagas' disease: trends in immunological research and prospects for immunoprophylaxis. Bulletin of the World Health Organization 57, 697-710.

Teixeira, A.R.L., Teixeira, M.L. and Santos-Buch, C.A. (1975). The immunology of experimental Chagas' disease. IV. Production of lesions in rabbits similar to those of chronic Chagas' disease in man. American Journal of Pathology 80, 163-178.

Tibayrenc, M., Cariou, M.L. and Solignac, M. (1981). Interprétation génétique des zymogrammes de flagellés des genres *Trypanosoma* et *Leishmania*. Compte rendu hebdomonadaire des Séances de l'Académie des Sciences 292, 623-625.

Urribarri, R.S. and Soto, S.T. de (1976). Consideraciones sobre aspectos epidemiologicos, de diagnostico y alteraciones eletrocard-iograficas mas frecuentes en 150 casos de enfermedad de Chagas cronica. Kasmera 5, 259-275.

World Health Organization (1980). Research on Chagas's disease. Bulletin of the World Health Organization 58, 574-575.

CHAPTER 2
Trypanosomiasis in the Absence of Tsetse

E.A. Wells

18, The Croft,
Sudbury, Suffolk,
CO10 6HP.

2.1. Introduction

The relationship between tsetse flies and trypanosomiasis of man and animals was first recognised at the end of the last century (Bruce 1895). Trypanosomes were first thought to be transmitted without multiplication or development in tsetse flies, being carried only passively on their mouth parts. This hypothesis of 'mechanical' (non-cyclical) transmission survived even after cyclical transmission in tsetse was demonstrated (Kleine 1909).

Infections of trypanosomes normally transmitted by tsetse in the apparent absence of tsetse have been reported from the African continent from the beginning of the century (*e.g.* Cazalbou 1905), and although many such allegations have since been discredited (Wells 1972), episodes are still reported (*e.g.* Tibayrenc and Gruvel 1977; Aeregan and Duwallet 1980). Mechanical transmission by haematophagous diptera other than tsetse is accepted as an explanation by most authors. This belief was reinforced by Hoare (1947, 1957), who theorized that *Trypanosoma vivax* established itself in Mauritius and the New World by adapting entirely to mechanical transmission. Hoare considered that *T. evansi* originated similarly from *T. brucei*, resulting in global spread of the infection.

The present article describes and compares the available epidemiological knowledge of *T. vivax* in Colombia and of *T. evansi* in north Vietnam, and uses it to discuss the hypothesis of non-cyclic, mechanical transmission. The nomenclature *Trypanosoma vivax viennei* and *T. brucei evansi* is used, as suggested by the international committee of 1976 (Anonymous 1978).

2.2. Epidemiology of *Trypanosoma vivax viennei* in Colombia

2.2.1. History

The historical background was described by Wells, Betancourt and
Page (1970). The movement of infected cattle from Senegal to the
Antilles in 1830 is surmised to have introduced the parasite to the
New World. The first introduction to Colombia probably occurred about
100 years later, associated with the importation of zebu cattle from
Venezuela through the port of Cartagena on the Caribbean coast. An
important mortality was recorded at the time in the indigenous cattle
with which they came in contact. In later years further episodes of
disease attributed to trypanosomiasis occurred in Colombia associated
with movements of cattle southwards from the north coast. A firm
belief was established amongst veterinarians and farmers that *T. vivax*
was an important pathogen causing a wasting syndrome and death.
Colloquial names were given to the infection - 'secadera', 'huequera'
and 'caucho hueco'. This belief, based on extrapolation from the
African situation, was challenged only by some sporadic work starting
in 1967. Serological work using the indirect fluorescent antibody
test (IFAT) was carried out between 1974 and 1978 (Platt and Adams
1976; Wells, Ramirez and Betancourt in press).

2.2.2. Geographical distribution, prevalence and incidence

Using IFAT, antibodies to *T. vivax viennei* have been found in loca-
tions representing 50% of the tropical and subtropical areas of
Colombia and 75% of the principal cattle areas of the country. When
the complementary evidence of positive blood smears is added, a reasonable assumption can be made that the trypanosome is distributed
throughout all tropical and subtropical Colombia. The IFAT also
indicated a wide variation in the percentage of positive animals between herds. Moreover, on the few occasions where herds had been
examined two or more times, significant fluctuations in the percentage
of positive animals occurred with time.

The best recorded information came from the tropical eastern plains
of Colombia. In order to set up a large scale beef production experiment, 340 cattle were purchased from several ranches. They were taken
from free range on flat plains intersected by gallery forests, to a
fenced situation allowing no contact with forest. On arrival, 44% of
cattle were serologically positive. Examination of the same sample of
animals (91) on 22 occasions over a period of 56 months showed an
irregular regression in the number of positive animals from 44% to nil.

In the same area of Colombia, 20 random serum samples from adult
cattle were examined, from each of 18 unfenced herds, twice with an
interval of 18 months. Whereas the overall figure of animals positive
showed no significant difference (53 and 50.8%), significant changes
in status appeared to occur in individual herds. The two herds with
the greatest changes showed an increase from 15 to 45% in one and a
decrease from 70 to 50% in the other.

The possibility of natural infections occurring in wild animals or any domestic animal other than cattle has not been examined.

2.2.3. Evidence relating to transmission

Dissections of diptera feeding from parasitaemic cattle in the field have failed to reveal any suspicion of infection with a salivarian trypanosome. The most important available evidence relates to movement of infected cattle. Such movements are alleged to have brought the infection from Africa, first to the Antilles and then to the continent of South America. The hypothesis is supported by evidence at the herd level. Betancourt (1978) followed sequences of clinical episodes which were all associated either with the transfer of cattle from herd to herd, or with infected herds coming into contact with susceptible herds.

2.4.4. Interpretation of data

The trypanosome appears to be distributed throughout the tropical and subtropical areas of Colombia, with variations in prevalence between herds, and variations in incidence in individual herds. The hypothesis can be made that the level of challenge varies, allowing herds to become susceptible to reinfection. Most reinfections are symptomless but, where clinical episodes occur, they may be related to the intensity of challenge and the breed of animal.

2.2.5. Economic impact

In the laboratory, clinical symptoms can be easily provoked in susceptible calves and goats (Daley 1971; Betancourt 1978). In the field, the wasting syndrome attributed to the trypanosome is now accepted as being primarily nutritional in origin (CIAT 1976). If a disease is involved in the complex, it is more likely to be anaplasmosis. However, clinical episodes of disease associated with *T. vivax* are known to occur sporadically, but their frequency has not been determined. They have been observed in both *Bos taurus* and *Bos indicus* breeds but the evidence indicates that *Bos taurus* breeds are more susceptible with acute episodes occurring in dairy cattle (Betancourt and Wells 1979).

2.3. Epidemiology of *Trypanosoma brucei evansi* in North Vietnam

2.3.1. History

The earliest evidence is given by Blanchard (1888), who described a disease in mules imported by the French Army. The disease could originally have spread from China following the introduction of the trypanosome in military animals imported by Anglo-Indian troops. Since these early days, farmers in the north of Vietnam are said to have been aware of trypanosomiasis as a disease.

The Department of Veterinary Services first recognized trypanosomiasis of buffalo (*Bubalus bubalis*) as a serious problem in the Red

River delta in 1954. At this time large numbers of buffalo were being
imported from the mountains to replace losses which had occurred
during the war of independence. The position worsened by 1978 when
not only were stocks of drugs finished but serious flooding meant that
rice fields had to be cultivated twice, causing severe work stress for
the depleted working buffalo population.

2.3.2. Geographical distribution, prevalence, incidence

The area affected by the problem comprises those provinces covering
the delta of the Red River (altitude 3-5 m), the mountains immediately
surrounding the delta (1100-1500 m), and the midlands interposed between the delta and the mountains (200-400 m). Clinical episodes of
trypanosomiasis have been described in three situations: in buffalo
in the mountains; in mountain buffalo when they reach the plain; and
in buffalo indigenous to the plain.

In the years 1970 to 1973 surveys for the trypanosome were carried
out by the Department of Veterinary Services. Two thousand buffalo
were sampled from each of the mountain, midland and delta areas.
Using blood smears and laboratory animal inoculation, 10-15% of mountain buffalo were found infected relative to the areas sampled, 10%
in the midlands and 60% in the delta.

The clinical episodes in the mountains are said to be associated with
spring, with the majority occurring at the highest altitudes. In the
delta plains they occur at any time of the year, but predominantly in
winter and spring.

Prevalence and incidence in other domesticated animals is unknown.
One acute episode has been described in cattle in the mountains.
Cattle, horses and dogs in the delta are known to be infected, but
acute clinical episodes do not occur. Pigs have never been sampled
in the field, but experimental infections are symptomless with parasitaemias detectable for a maximum of 4 months.

2.3.3. Evidence relating to transmission

The Department of Veterinary Services carried out a survey of 9000
biting flies and ticks between January 1967 and July 1968. The range
and abundance of species found in the mountains and midlands greatly
exceeded those found in the plains. Transmission appears to occur
easily when infected and susceptible buffalo are mixed.

2.3.4. Interpretation of data

The situation can be explained by the difference in the prevalence
of infection between the plains and the mountain areas. There is a
high prevalence of infection in the plains and clinical episodes occur
under stress of work, malnutrition and adverse weather. The period
when trypanosomiasis is principally diagnosed is December to March.
The maximum work load for buffalo extends from October to March,

coinciding with the coldest weather and poorest feed availability.

The prevalence of infection in mountain buffalo is relatively lower. Clinical episodes may more often involve animals with no immunity and are therefore more acute in their manifestation. Clinical episodes in the Government stations probably result from the mixing of carrier and susceptible animals from different areas. When taken to the plains, susceptible mountain cattle receive a severe challenge from trypanosomiasis, superimposed on the stress of trekking.

2.3.5. Economic impact

Least information is available for clinical episodes in mountain buffalo, but they are said to be acute with high mortality. The mortality in the government collecting stations, organized to despatch replacement buffalo to the delta, is also considered by veterinary staff to be due primarily or solely to trypanosomiasis. The mortality (50-90%) in mountain buffalo on arrival in the plain is considered by staff to be due to trypanosomiasis aggravated by the stress of travel. Episodes in buffalo indigenous to the plain are less acute, with a maximum mortality of 10% blamed on trypanosomiasis imposed on starvation, overwork and cold weather. In 1978, the Department of Veterinary Services stated that 20 600 buffalo died of trypanosomiasis in the Red River delta, representing 3.1% of the total buffalo population.

No information exists on the influence of trypanosomiasis on abortion rate, loss of weight and loss of work. However, sufficient is known to state that trypanosomiasis as a complication to starved and overworked animals is an important cause of annual wastage in working buffalo. This is a critical factor in an area dependent on draught buffalo for crop production.

2.4. Discussion

These two brief epidemiological descriptions involve two different species of salivarian trypanosome against different social and agricultural backgrounds. Both trypanosomes are being transmitted in the absence of tsetse fly. The global distribution of *T. brucei evansi* has been well described and delineated for many years (Hoare 1972). Similar information for *T. vivax viennei* has only relatively recently been available. Serological evidence from IFAT has shown that the distribution in the New World may extend between the same latitudes as that of *T. vivax vivax* in the Old World, from Paraguay in the south to El Salvador in the north (Wells, Betancourt and Ramirez 1977). The evidence is supported by the demonstration of the parasite on blood slides from Panama, Colombia, Venezuela, Guyana, Surinam, French Guiana, northern Brazil, Ecuador and Peru.

The wide distribution of both trypanosomes appears to have been effected by the movement of infected animals into new countries and continents. This has been reflected in the descriptions of the Colombian and Vietnamese situations where the mixing of infected and

susceptible animals can provoke new infections. The inference is that
there are ubiquitous vectors, and the concept of mechanical, non-cyclic,
transmission is at once reasonable. However, there are fundamental
questions yet to be answered if the trypanosomiases are examined on a
world basis. Some subjects for investigation are: whether some trypanosome species or populations are more amenable to non-cyclical
transmission than others; whether some arthropods, particularly dipteran
species, are more capable of mechanical transmission than others; the
economics of vector control outside the distribution of tsetse fly;
the epidemiological importance of such non-cyclical transmission within the distribution of tsetse fly in Africa; and the dynamics of
mechanical transmission. The last question is basic to the credibility
of this mode of transmission.

If the level of parasitaemia in a carrier animal is considered, together with the amount of blood that may remain in the proboscis of a
biting fly disturbed at feeding, then the number of biting flies
needed to deliver an infective dose to a susceptible animal could be
very large. The largest number would be required in those circumstances
where host defences are overwhelmed and a clinical episode ensues.
If no multiplication of trypanosomes occurs in the vectors, then at
least some mechanism for extracting and concentrating trypanosomes in
probosces during feeding on parasitaemic blood can be postulated.

With the exception of venereal infection caused by *T. brucei equiperdum*,
the lack of epidemiological information on the transmission of salivarian trypanosomes in the absence of tsetse can in part be blamed on
a lack of techniques usable in the field. The present availability
of serological tests and complementary techniques for detecting low
parasitaemias means that the field conditions within which transmission
occurs can be be better defined, and entomological work better oriented.
However, investigation of economic loss from *T. brucei evansi* and *T.
vivax viennei* may have a low research priority in countries with
limited laboratory resource. An argument can be made for an international programme to examine the existence and relative importance
of all modes of salivarian trypanosome transmission in the absence of
tsetse.

The most rewarding sites for investigation would probably be in South
America, where transmission of *T. brucei evansi* and *T. vivax viennei*
may be studied in the same or adjacent localities. The relationship
of *T. vivax viennei* to both *T. vivax vivax* and *T. vivax uniforme* of
Africa should be early examined by analysis of isoenzymes, in the
same way that the relationship of *T. brucei evansi* and *T. brucei brucei*
has already been established (Gibson *et al.* 1980). Work on *T. brucei
evansi*, a species more amenable to handling in the laboratory, may
indicate lines of approach to *T. vivax viennei*, and combined study of
both could indicate optimal lines of investigation within the distribution of tsetse in the Old World.

Even after nearly 90 years of tsetse and trypanosomiasis research,
the mode of transmission of salivarian trypanosomes in the absence of

tsetse is still on the frontier of knowledge.

Acknowledgements

The work recorded from Colombia was carried out as part of the animal health programme of the Centro Internacional de Agricultura Tropical (CIAT), Cali. The information from Vietnam was collected during a consultancy carried out by the author on behalf of the Animal Production and Health Division, Food and Agriculture Organization, Rome, following an earlier visit by Dr P. Finelle. Thanks are due to the Director of Veterinary Services, Vietnam, for permission to quote from Departmental archives.

2.5. References

Aeregan G. and Duwallet, G. (1980). A focus of human African trypanosomiasis without tsetse flies. Médecine tropicale 10, 367–371.

Anonymous (1978). Proposals for the nomenclature of salivarian trypanosomes and for the maintenance of reference collections. Bulletin of the World Health Organization 56, 467–480.

Betancourt, A. (1978). Studies on the epidemiology and economic importance of *Trypanosoma vivax* Ziemann, 1905 in Colombia. Ph. D. dissertation, Texas A. and M. University.

Betancourt A. and Wells, E.A. (1979). Pérdidas económicas en un brote de tripanosomiasis causada por *Trypanosoma vivax*. Revista Acovez 3, 6–9.

Blanchard, R. (1888). Étude sur une maladie spéciale des mulets importés au Tonkin pour le service de l'armée et considérations sur l'acclimatement de l'espèce chevaline en Extrême Orient. Bulletin de la Société Centrale de Médecine Vétérinaire 42, 694–702.

Bruce, D. (1895). Preliminary report on the tsetse fly disease or nagana in Zululand. Bennett and Davis, Durban.

Cazalbou, L. (1905). Le Macina foyer permanent de trypanosomiase. Comptes rendus des séances de la Société de Biologie 58, 564–565.

CIAT (1976). Animal Health section: production systems for beef cattle. Centro Internacional de Agricultura Tropical, Annual Report for 1975, pp. A39–A40. Cali, Colombia.

Daley, C.A. (1971). A sequential study of the pathogenesis of disease caused by *Trypanosoma vivax* in experimentally infected calves, utilising clinical, pathological, histopathological and immunofluorescent techniques. M. Sc. thesis, Texas A. and M. University.

Gibson, W.C., Marshall, T.F. de C. and Godfrey, D.G. (1980). Numerical analysis of enzyme polymorphism: a new approach to the epidemiology and taxonomy of trypanosomes of the subgenus *Trypanozoon*. Advances in Parasitology 18, 175–246.

24

Hoare, C.A. (1947). Tsetse borne trypanosomiases outside their natural boundaries. Annales de la Société belge de Médecine Tropicale 27, Supplement, 267-277.

Hoare, C.A. (1957). The spread of African trypanosomes beyond their natural range. Zeitschrift für Tropenmedizin und Parasitologie 8, 157-161.

Hoare, C.A. (1972). The trypanosomes of mammals. Blackwell Scientific Publications, Oxford and Edinburgh.

Kleine, F. (1909). Positive Infektionsversuche mit *Trypanosoma brucei* durch *Glossina palpalis*. Deutsche medizinische Wochenschrift 35, 409-470 and 1257-1260.

Platt, K.B. and Adams, L.G. (1976). Evaluation of the indirect fluorescent antibody test for detecting *Trypanosoma vivax* in South American cattle. Research in Veterinary Science 21, 53-58.

Tibayrenc, R. and Gruvel, J. (1977). La campagne de lutte contre les glossines dans la bassin du lac Tchad. II.Contrôle de l'assainissement glossinaire. Revue d'Élevage et de Médécine Vétérinaire des Pays Tropicaux 30, 31-39.

Wells, E.A. (1972). The importance of mechanical transmission in the epidemiology of nagana: a review. Tropical Animal Health and Production 4, 74-78.

Wells, E.A., Betancourt, A., and Page, W.A. (1970). The epidemiology of bovine trypanosomiasis in Colombia. Tropical Animal Health and Production 2, 111-125.

Wells, E.A., Betancourt, A., and Ramirez, L.E. (1977). Serological evidence for the geographical distribution of *Trypanosoma vivax* in the New World. Transactions of the Royal Society of Tropical Medicine and Hygiene 71, 448-449.

Wells, E.A., Ramirez, L.E., and Betancourt, A. (in press). *Trypanosoma vivax* in Colombia: interpretation of field results using the indirect fluorescent antibody test. Tropical Animal Health and Production.

CHAPTER 3
Trypanosomes in African Wild Mammals

D. Mehlitz

Abteilung für Veterinärmedizin,
Bernhard-Nocht-Institut für Schiffs- und Tropenkrankheiten,
Bernhard-Nocht-Strasse 74,
D-2000 Hamburg 4.

3.1. Introduction

In this paper I try to relate experiences and problems resulting
from field and laboratory work in Botswana, Upper Volta and Liberia,
to earlier investigations carried out mainly in eastern and southern
Africa, and to point out those things we do not know rather than those
we think we know. One may ask, why are we interested in trypanosomes
in game animals at all? In my opinion, the subject is important for
two reasons: (1) wild animals are generally believed to be 'resistant'
to trypanosomiasis, and/or to show different levels of 'trypanotolerance', manifested as reduced susceptibility to the pathogenic effects
of trypanosome infection (Murray *et al*. 1979 and in press); and (2)
the importance of wild animal species as reservoir hosts for trypanosomes infecting domestic animals and man, which is related to their
resistance and tolerance. Work on both aspects is a challenge to
everyone concerned with trypanosomiasis and the epidemiology of the
disease.

3.2. Susceptibility to infection

Different degrees of susceptibility to trypanosomes of the subgenera
Trypanozoon, *Nannomonas* or *Duttonella* exist between various wild
mammalian species, as shown more than 20 years ago by Ashcroft *et al*.
(1959). This wide spectrum of susceptibilities ranges from the complete refractoriness of the baboon (*Papio* spp.) to the high susceptibility of Thomson's gazelle (*Gazella thomsonii*) with a fatal outcome
following experimentally induced *Trypanozoon* infections.

Most of the information available on trypanosomes and game comes
from reports of infection rates in various species and various localities. Speculations on the susceptibility of certain species are
based on these infection rates, which are only very rough estimates
and can be influenced by many factors such as vector density, season,

virulence of the trypanosome species in the study area and, to a great extent, different diagnostic methods used by the various investigators. Therefore, prevalence figures of trypanosome infection vary between 1.3% and 38.2%, and thus do not give very much information on the susceptibility of different species. This is illustrated by Table 1, summarizing the detectable trypanosome infections in wild animals examined last year (1980) in Upper Volta. The limitations of results like these could be applicable to those published by other workers, for the reasons set out below.

3.3. Factors influencing infection rates

3.3.1. Availability of animals

The availability of animal species and the numbers examined are restricted mainly by the extreme difficulty of obtaining blood samples. That is to say, random sampling to obtain quantitative results from all species of interest is not feasible for the population in a given area. An outstanding result such as 47.5% parasitologically positive kob is very exciting; but it is not comparable with results from species of which only a few samples could be examined, and from which insufficient evidence is therefore available regarding susceptibility to infection, such as the duikers or the buffalo in this example (Table 1: scientific names of wild mammals are given in Table 2). Further, species showing low prevalences of infection do not necessarily have low susceptibility. They may be infected, with high parasitaemias, but then die within a short period or be killed by predators because of weakness, and thus be unavailable for examination.

3.3.2. Diagnostic methods

Another important reason for limited information is the diagnostic method itself. Even if the most sensitive parasitological method available, such as the mini-anion exchange-centrifugation method, the haematocrit centrifugation technique or rodent subinoculation, is used quite a number of cryptic infections are inevitably missed due to insufficient sensitivity. Parasitological methods should be supplemented by serological diagnostic techniques, which were applied only exceptionally in the past (Binz and Allsopp 1972; Dräger and Mehlitz 1978). Table 1 also shows the number of animals in which circulating anti-trypanosomal antibodies were detected which more accurately reflects true susceptibilities. But here again, conclusions regarding the true infection rate at the time of examination are doubtful, as the circulating antibodies indicate only a previous contact of the host with the parasite. Common serological tests, such as immunofluorescence or the enzyme-linked immunosorbent assay (ELISA), have the disadvantage that normally a specific anti-host conjugate is not available for the different game animal species. This could be overcome by using an immunofluorescent complement fixation test or the immunoperoxidase-complement fixation test, which are independent of specific anti-game conjugate (Perié et al. 1975; Hörchner et al. 1979). A diagnostic technique specific at the level of trypanosome species,

Table 1. Trypanosome infections of wild mammals in Upper Volta

| Species | Number examined | PARASITOLOGY Number of infections with | | | | | SEROLOGY |
		Trypanozoon spp.	Nannomonas spp.	Duttonella spp.	Unidentified spp. (including Megatrypanum)	No. of infected animals	Number of animals with anti-Trypanosoma antibody
Kob	40	13 (32.7%)	3	4	8	19	25/39
Hartebeest	26	2	1	1	1	4	10/25
Oribi	15	–	–	1	4	4	9/13
Bushbuck	4	2	3	1	1	3	3/3
Warthog	14	–	1	–	–	1	2/14
Waterbuck	3	1	–	–	–	1	3/3
Roan antelope	3	–	1	–	1	2	3/3
Buffalo	2	–	–	–	–	0	2/2
Grey duiker	4	–	–	–	–	0	4/4
Red duiker	2	–	–	–	–	0	2/2
TOTAL	113					34 (30.1%)	63/108 (58.3%)

28

Table 2. Scientific names of wild mammals

Buffalo	*Syncerus caffer*
Bushbuck	*Tragelaphus scriptus*
Duiker, grey	*Sylvicapra grimmia*
Duiker, red	*Cephalophus harveyi*
Hartebeest	*Alcelaphus buselaphus*
Kob	*Kobus kob*
Oribi	*Ourebia ourebi*
Roan antelope	*Hippotragus equinus*
Warthog	*Phacochoerus aethiopicus*
Waterbuck	*Kobus defassa*

would be very valuable but has not yet been developed.

3.3.3. Host preferences of *Glossina*

Speculations on susceptibility usually consider the host preferences of the tsetse flies (*Glossina* spp.) in the study area. It is well known that warthogs are among those species from which a very high percentage of blood meals is identified in tsetse, but trypanosome infections in warthogs are relatively rare. On the other hand, feeds from waterbuck are almost never identified by blood meal analysis, but these antelope show a high prevalence rate (Ashcroft *et al*. 1959). Is it therefore justifiable to conclude that waterbuck are outstandingly susceptible to trypanosome infection? Could the blood meal analysis be a misleading indicator, not considering the possibility that the flies only probe and do not feed for some reason?

3.3.4. Age of host

The age of the host may also influence the infection rate found in individuals even within one species. Figure 1 shows parasitologically proven diagnoses and antibody levels in buffalo of different age groups: less than 1 year (n=85), 1-3 years (n=74), 4-7 years (n=128) and over 7 years (n=211). Buffalo calves under one year old were rarely found infected - only 1.4% - and were generally serologically negative. The infection might have been suppressed by innate resistance or by transfer of colostral antibodies. In the age group of 1-3 years, a significant increase of parasitologically positive animals was detected (34.4%). As the resistance of the calves waned, patent infections developed, and these might have induced the production of humoral antibodies. In other words, the innate relative resistance of the calf was possibly followed by a state of premunity. The effect of this premunity might be seen in the steady decrease of patent infections in the older buffalo, in which, at the same time, anti-

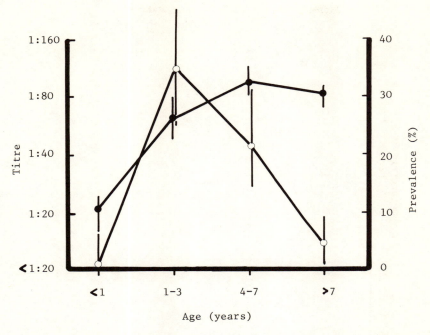

Figure 1. Relation between age of buffalo (*Syncerus caffer*), IFAT
   titre (solid circles) and prevalence of trypanosome infection (open
   circles); vertical bars indicate 95% confidence limits. (Redrawn,
   with permission, from Dräger and Mehlitz 1978, Tropenmedizin und
   Parasitologie, vol. 29, pp. 223-233.)

bodies persisted.

3.3.5. Infectivity of trypanosomes

I have not so far touched on the possible alteration of infectivity
of the trypanosome population and its influence on prevalence rates.
In Botswana we were, surprisingly, unable to infect mice with *Trypanozoon* from any of 7 infected buffalo, but we succeeded with *Trypanozoon*
from 8 of 9 infected lechwe (*Kobus leche*) in the same area. Is this
loss of infectivity due to long periods spent previously in the ungu-
late hosts, which Duke (1937) suggested, long ago, might account for
loss of infectivity to man by *Trypanozoon* species? Alternatively,
may the infectivity be increased by quick passages in areas of high
tsetse challenge, if one assumes that the flies prefer lechwe to
buffalo? Recently the total loss of rodent infectivity by *T. brucei*
and *T. rhodesiense* clones after incubation with serum of an eland
(*Taurotragus oryx*) was reported (Rickman 1981; Rickman *et al*. 1981).
However, this very interesting observation cannot be generalized to
permit the conclusion that certain game species have trypanosomicidal

Table 3. Enzyme profiles and sensitivity to human serum of 15 *Trypanozoon* stocks from wild and domestic animals and man in Upper Volta.

Host	Serum sensitivity results*	Enzyme profiles**						
		ALAT	ASAT	ICD	PEP2	PEP1	PGM	ME
1 hartebeest	S							
2 domestic pig	S, +							
1 ox	+++	II	I	II	I	II	II	I
1 man	+							
1 kob	+							
1 domestic pig	+							
1 man	+++	II	I	II	I	II	II	XV
1 kob	S							
1 dog	S	II	I	II	I	I	II	I
6 domestic pig	4S, 2+							
1 kob	+++	II	I	II	I	II	II	XI
1 waterbuck	S	II	I	II	I	VI	II	I
2 kob	S, +							
1 bushbuck	S	II	I	II	I	VI	II	XV
1 ox	+++							
1 hartebeest	S	II	I	II	I	VI	II	XXII

Table 3. (Continued).

Host	Serum sensitivity results*	Enzyme profiles**						
		ALAT	ASAT	ICD	PEP2	PEP1	PGM	ME
1 kob	S	II	I	II	I	XI	II	I
1 kob	+++	VIII	I	II	I	I	II	I
1 domestic pig	S							
2 kob	+++,+++	VIII	I	II	I	I	V	I
1 kob	S	X	I	II	I	VI	II	XV
1 kob	S	X	I	II	I	XI	II	I

* Blood incubation infectivity test: +++ = highly resistant to human serum; + = subresistant;
  S = sensitive.

** ALAT = alanine aminotransferase (EC2.6.1.2); ASAT = aspartate aminotransferase (EC2.6.1.1);
   ICD = isocitrate dehydrogenase (EC1.1.1.42); PEP2 and PEP1 = two peptidases (EC3.4.11), with
   substrates L-leucyl-L-alanine and L-leucylglycylglycine, respectively; PGM = phosphoglucomutase
   (EC2.7.5.1); ME = "malic" enzyme (EC1.1.1.40).

serum components, as the same species, the eland, has been demonstrated to harbour *T. brucei* naturally and experimentally (Ashcroft *et al.* 1959).

3.3.6. Trypanotolerance

If trypanotolerance is basically under genetic control with genetic diversity within one breed (Cox and Cross 1979), and this phenomenon is the result of selection, the knowledge obtained from experiments – in which 1-5 animals of a species are examined for their susceptibility to infection – or from field studies, is very limited indeed. Immuno-logical mechanisms influencing trypanotolerance, as discussed for different breeds of cattle and mice by Murray *et al.* (1979 and in press), Morrison *et al.* (1978) and Morrison and Murray (1979), need further attention. Study of mechanisms governing trypanotolerance – and therefore susceptibility – should be concentrated on experiments with game animals kept in captivity in a tsetse free environment under controlled conditions, with the particular aim of developing a model for certain domestic animal breeds, nowadays propagated very intens-ively to increase animal protein sources mainly in the humid areas of western and central Africa.

3.3.7. Pathogenicity of trypanosomes

Very little information is yet available on the behaviour of tryp-anosomes in game animals, particularly concerning infectivity or pathogenicity for a new host. It was shown recently, in Kenya, that clinically healthy buffalo exhibited *T. vivax* infections, isolates of which were very pathogenic for cattle (Olubayo 1979). More intensive studies, mainly on the subgenus *Trypanozoon*, attempted a character-ization by testing sensitivity to normal human serum as an estimate of potential infectivity to man (Rickman and Robson 1970; Hawking 1976a, b; Mehlitz 1978) or by carrying out isoenzyme electrophoresis (Godfrey and Kilgour 1976; Gibson *et al.* 1978, 1980). Comparisons of stocks isolated from game with those derived from domestic animals or from man demonstrated identical zymodemes. Table 3 shows that zymodemes found in stocks from a hartebeest and a kob had their exact counterparts in stocks from domestic animals and man. These results, together with others and our previous observations in Liberia, indicate that gambiense sleeping sickness is a zoonosis (Mehlitz 1977, 1978; Gibson *et al.* 1978, 1980; Mehlitz *et al.* in press). Another signifi-cant observation, on trypanosomes with alanine aminotransferase pattern II as a marker, was the variability in response to normal human serum, even with stocks originating from man. Again, the question is raised (Hawking 1977, 1979) whether or not partially resistant trypanosomes from animals are potentially infective to man; perhaps only after successfully infecting man or establishing a man-fly-man cycle do they become highly resistant to human serum. At present, in West Africa at least, the value of a negative result in the blood incubation infectivity test (*i.e.*, serum sensitivity) as an indicator of lack of infectivity to man, must be regarded as doubtful; in all likelihood, however, a positive result (*i.e.* resistance to human serum) indicates human infectivity.

Further intensive studies aimed at the intrinsic characterization
of trypanosomes of *Trypanozoon* and, especially, of *Duttonella* and
Nannomonas, may provide valuable information about infectivity and
pathogenicity of stocks originating from various epidemiological
situations in Africa.

3.4. Conclusions

Finally, I wish to stress the need to intensify studies on game
animals, firstly to clarify the local epidemiology and epizootiology
of trypanosomiasis, and secondly to provide experimental animal models
to study the various degrees of trypanotolerance.

However, work with wild animals is getting more and more difficult
in Africa. For political reasons, in many African countries there is
a general hunting prohibition which applies partly also to the immob-
ilization of animals. It will need enormous effort to convince
officials to provide licences. Further, a project on game trypanosomiasis and the procedure of getting samples of wild animals is extremely
time consuming and costly. Wildlife experts are rare. Experience
from game parks in East Africa, where game is abundant, is not trans-
ferable to West African savannah areas with much less game, or - least
of all - to rain forest areas from which information on game trypanosomiasis is completely lacking.

Therefore, in my opinion, the inevitably limited resources of funds,
manpower and expertise should be concentrated by attempting interdisciplinary cooperation covering all aspects of epidemiology in a
small number of integrated projects, rather than being wasted on
isolated schemes.

3.5. References

Ashcroft, M.T., Burtt, E. and Fairbairn, H. (1959). The experimental
infection of some African wild animals with *Trypanosoma rhodesiense*,
T. brucei and *T. congolense*. Annals of Tropical Medicine and
Parasitology 53, 147-161.

Binz, G. and Allsopp, R. (1972). Preliminary observations on the use
of the latex agglutination test for detecting circulating trypanosomal antibodies in game animals in the Lambwe Valley. Bulletin of
the World Health Organization 47, 769-772.

Cox, F.E.G. and Cross, G.A.M. (1979). Infections. Discussion summary,
in Pathogenicity of Trypanosomes (edited by G. Losos and A. Chouinard),
pp. 89-90. International Development Research Centre, Ottawa.
(Publication number 1DRC-132e.)

Dräger, N. and Mehlitz, D. (1978). Investigations on the prevalence
of trypanosome carriers and the antibody response in wildlife in
northern Botswana. Tropenmedizin und Parasitologie 29, 223-233.

34

Duke, H.L. (1937). Studies on the effect on *T. gambiense* and *T. rhodesiense* of prolonged maintenance in mammals other than man; with special reference to the power of these trypanosomes to infect man. V. The effect of prolonged maintenance away from man on the infectivity of *T. rhodesiense* for man. Parasitology 29, 12-34.

Gibson, W., Mehlitz, D., Lanham, S.M. and Godfrey, D.G. (1978). The identification of *Trypanosoma brucei gambiense* in Liberian pigs and dogs by isoenzymes and by resistance to human plasma. Tropenmedizin und Parasitologie 29, 335-345.

Gibson, W.C., Marshall, T.F. de C. and Godfrey, D.G. (1980). Numerical analysis of enzyme polymorphism: a new approach to the epidemiology and taxonomy of trypanosomes of the subgenus *Trypanozoon*. Advances in Parasitology 18, 175-246.

Godfrey, D.G. and Kilgour, V. (1976). Enzyme electrophoresis in characterizing the causative organism of Gambian trypanosomiasis. Transactions of the Royal Society of Tropical Medicine and Hygiene 70, 219-224.

Hawking, F. (1976a). The resistance to human plasma of *Trypanosoma brucei*, *T. rhodesiense* and *T. gambiense*. I. Analysis of the composition of trypanosome strains. Transactions of the Royal Society of Tropical Medicine and Hygiene 70, 504-512.

Hawking, F. (1976b). The resistance to human plasma of *Trypanosoma brucei*, *T. rhodesiense* and *T. gambiense*. II. Survey of strains from East Africa and Nigeria. Transactions of the Royal Society of Tropical Medicine and Hygiene 70, 513-520.

Hawking, F. (1977). The resistance to human plasma of *Trypanosoma brucei*, *T. rhodesiense* and *T. gambiense*. III. Clones of two plasma-resistant strains. Transactions of the Royal Society of Tropical Medicine and Hygiene 71, 427-430.

Hawking, F. (1979). The action of human serum upon *Trypanosoma brucei*. Protozoological Abstracts 3, 199-206.

Hörchner, F., Bofenschen, F. and Zander, B. (1979). Zur serologischen Differenzierung von *Trypanosoma brucei-*, *T. congolense-* und *T. vivax-*infektionen. Tropenmedizin und Parasitologie 30, 265-273.

Mehlitz, D. (1977). The behaviour in the blood incubation infectivity test of four *Trypanozoon* strains isolated from pigs in Liberia. Transactions of the Royal Society of Tropical Medicine and Hygiene 71, 86.

Mehlitz, D. (1978). Untersuchungen zur Empfänglichkeit von *Mastomys natalensis* für *Trypanosoma (Trypanozoon) brucei gambiense*. Tropenmedizin und Parasitologie 29, 101-107.

Mehlitz, D., Zillmann, U., Scott, C.M. and Godfrey, D.G. (in press). Epidemiological studies on the animal reservoir of Gambian sleeping sickness. Part III. Characterization of *Trypanozoon* stocks by isoenzymes and sensitivity to human serum. Tropenmedizin und Parasitologie.

Morrison, W.I. and Murray, M. (1979). *Trypanosoma congolense*: inheritance of susceptibility to infection in inbred strains of mice. Experimental Parasitology 48, 364-374.

Morrison, W.I., Roelants, G.E., Mayor-Withey, K.S. and Murray, M. (1978). Susceptibility of inbred strains of mice to *Trypanosoma congolense*: correlation with changes in spleen lymphocyte populations. Clinical and Experimental Immunology 32, 25-40.

Murray, M., Morrison, W.I., Murray, R.K., Clifford, D.J. and Trail, J.C.M. (1979). Trypanotolerance: a review. World Animal Review 31, 2-12.

Murray, M., Morrison, W.I. and Whitelaw, D.D. (in press). Host susceptibility to African trypanosomiasis: trypanotolerance. Advances in Parasitology 21.

Olubayo, R. (1979). Trypanosomiasis of game animals, in Pathogenicity of Trypanosomes (edited by G. Losos and A. Chouinard), pp. 87-88. International Development Research Centre, Ottawa. (Publication number 1DRC-132e.)

Perié, N.M., Tinnemans-Anggawidjaja, T. and Zwart, D. (1975). A refinement of the immunofluorescent complement fixation test for *Trypanosoma* infections. Tropenmedizin und Parasitologie 26, 399-404.

Rickman, L.R. (1981). The effects of some African game animal sera in the BIIT on the *Trypanosoma (Trypanozoon) brucei* species [sic] trypanosomes. Transactions of the Royal Society of Tropical Medicine and Hygiene 75, 122-123.

Rickman, L.R. and Robson, J. (1970). The testing of proven *Trypanosoma brucei* and *T. rhodesiense* strains by the blood incubation infectivity test. Bulletin of the World Health Organization 42, 911-916.

Rickman, L.R., Kolala, F. and Mwanza, S. (1981). Variation in the sensitivity of successive variable antigen types in a *Trypanosoma (Trypanozoon) brucei* subspecies clone to some African game animal sera. Acta Tropica 38, 115-124.

CHAPTER 4
Diversity Within *Trypanosoma congolense*

D.G. Godfrey

MRC External Staff,
Department of Medical Protozoology,
London School of Hygiene and Tropical Medicine,
Winches Farm Field Station,
395 Hatfield Road,
St Albans, Hertfordshire, AL4 OXQ.

4.1. Introduction

This paper puts forward evidence that *Trypanosoma congolense* is a collection of widely diverse organisms and not just a simple species within the subgenus *Nannomonas*. It is essential to realize this when dealing with its much neglected epidemiology; experimental descriptions of a few easily maintained laboratory specimens are not necessarily applicable to the variety of organisms which differ remarkably in such behavioural properties as infectivity, host range and pathogenicity, just as much as the similar but well recognized differences within *T. brucei*. In addition, *T. congolense* appears to be especially prone to develop persistently drug-resistant forms (see Leach and Roberts 1981), but, important as this propensity is, only naturally occurring diversity will be considered.

4.2. Isoenzyme characterization

Epidemiology depends on the accurate identification of behaviourally different organisms, and, in the past few years, we have been using isoenzyme electrophoresis extensively to identify subspecies of *Trypanozoon* for epidemiological investigations (Godfrey and Kilgour 1976; Gibson *et al*. 1978, 1980; Mehlitz *et al*. in press). Young (1980) began similar work on *T. congolense* and, despite the difficulties of raising adequate parasitaemias, determined profiles of 12 enzymes in 78 stocks from all over Africa; most were freshly isolated and passaged only a few times. Each stock was identified by 20-34 characters, the isoenzyme bands that were manifestations of molecular polymorphism in nine enzymes; the remaining three enzymes were identical in every stock, showing the broad unity within the collection. Without going into detail or pretending that the problems of subspecific recognition within *Nannomonas* are entirely solved, I believe the findings are a progressive step in the right direction, giving some insight into the epidemiological significance of strains and illustrating the distinct genetic diversity in the species.

Following the computer method of Gibson *et al*. (1980) to establish the proportion of isoenzyme bands common between two stocks, degrees of relationship were built up and a dendrogram produced. The *T. congolense* stocks examined clearly fell into two major divisions, similar only at about the 20% level, with only three anomalous stocks. The interesting finding was that the division occurred between those stocks isolated from dry savannah areas and those from the humid coastal areas of West Africa; this suggests that the enzymic differences are fundamental, since the computer created the division solely on such differences, the provenance of the stocks being superimposed afterwards by ourselves. Gibson *et al*. (1980) reported a major geographic separation between East and West African *Trypanozoon* stocks, based on enzyme characterization. The obvious conjecture is that the *T. congolense* division is associated with transmission by the different tsetse species that inhabit the separate habitats. This must be proven experimentally but I have previously argued that enzyme modifications may be associated with adaptation to particular vectors (Godfrey 1979), while Miles *et al*. (1981) considered such an association possible between *T. cruzi* zymodemes and vectors.

However, any means of characterization can lead to wrong conclusions if too few samples from too few areas are compared using too few characters. I have already mentioned the three enzymes examined which did not vary electrophoretically among the 78 stocks, and which illustrated an underlying affinity. However, perhaps an insufficient number of samples was looked at. For example, threonine dehydrogenase was believed at first not to vary among the subgenus *Trypanozoon*; it was only after over 100 stocks were studied that rare variations in this enzyme were found, all from what may be a special kind of *T. brucei* occurring in parts of East Africa (Gibson *et al*. 1980). Thus care must be taken not to be categorical concerning the lack of variation in an enzyme until long experience justifies it. This holds true for any intrinsic character, including a morphological one, and acceptance of a so called distinguishing feature before wide assessment should be avoided.

Another enzyme studied in *T. congolense* was glyceraldehyde phosphate dehydrogenase (GAPDH), which had just two variations or patterns in contrast to the 18 patterns found with one of the peptidases; the other enzymes showing polymorphism had numbers between these two extremes. It was surprising how many of these different forms were found in one village (Table 1). Both molecular forms of GAPDH existed in the village, yet only one of the seven glucose phosphate isomerase (GPI) variations. Obviously taxonomic conclusions from a limited number of stocks in one area should not be reached without having a wider appreciation of the variation possible; the organisms are certainly different in the one area, but the epidemiological significance of each kind is difficult to assess without much wider information.

Table 1. *T. congolense*: number of patterns found for various enzymes
in 1 village compared with those seen throughout Africa (based on
data by Young 1980, adjusted to ignore differences between patterns
differing only in strength of certain component band activities).

| Enzymes* | No. of enzyme patterns seen: | |
	Keneba, The Gambia	Throughout Africa
GAPDH	2	2
ASAT	3	4
PGM	1	3
MDH	2	4
ALAT	3	5
ME	2	5
GPI	1	7
PEP 2	4	14
PEP 1	4	18

*GAPDH = glyceraldehyde phosphate dehydrogenase (EC 1.2.1.12),
ASAT = aspartate aminotransferase (EC 2.6.1.1), PGM = phosphogluco-
mutase (EC 2.7.5.1), MDH = malate dehydrogenase (EC 1.1.1.37),
ALAT = alanine aminotransferase (EC 2.6.1.2), ME = "malic" enzyme
(EC 1.1.1.40), GPI = glucose phosphate isomerase (EC 5.3.1.9),
PEP 2 and PEP 1 = two peptidases (EC 3.4.11), with substrates L-
leucyl-L-alanine and L-leucylglycylglycine respectively.

What is especially interesting is that the computer assessment of
isoenzyme relationships showed that most of the samples from various
places within The Gambia fell into two distinct groups, each group
with close internal affinities. Both kinds occurred in the village
mentioned in Table 1. Both were included in the major 'dry' zone
division, together with another clear geographical group, comprising
stocks almost entirely from eastern Africa. Again the computer con-
structed the groups according to enzyme profiles, independently of
the origins of the stocks. The significance of these further divisions
is uncertain, but provides a basis for future comparative studies with
defined stocks rather than those chosen haphazardly.

Any set of characters, not only isoenzymes, can be used to produce
a classification of use to epidemiologists. Although many more independent characters can now be used for identifying protozoa, they
will probably be only a small fraction of the total of similar characters within the cell; the enzymes examined are but a few of the many
hundreds in the trypanosome. Should then the enzymes that do not vary
in *T. congolense* be included in the analysis? Chance selection of
those common to the organisms weights the data towards greater

similarity; the classical numerical taxonomists believe these should
be excluded (Sneath and Sokal 1973). They also consider every variable
character of equal value, which means that every band of a highly
polymorphic enzyme, like the peptidases in *T. congolense*, has the same
significance as a band of a slightly polymorphic one. Again, such
problems must be considered whatever the means of characterization.

4.3. Differences in infectivity

For the reasons indicated above, many samples are necessary to
evaluate any set of characteristics, whether for epidemiology or taxonomy. But is every kind of *T. congolense* being examined? Up to now,
most characterizations or descriptions, whether biochemical or behavioural, have depended on the isolates being maintained in the laboratory.
Strong evidence exists, however, that certain kinds of *T. congolense*
are seldom isolated and hence are rarely studied, yet an adequate
characterization of all is essential for a full understanding of
epidemiology.

Among the early reports, Bruce *et al*. (1911) and Laveran and Mesnil
(1912) described a form, called *T. nanum* by them, which was not infective to rodents and dogs, while Peel and Chardome (1954a) also
described isolates from Zaire which would not infect mice. Many years
ago, one isolation maintained cyclically with some difficulty in
Nigeria infected only a few rats, which survived the infection with
extremely low parasitaemias (Godfrey 1961). This isolation infected
dogs via tsetse flies but did not kill them, unlike another stock
being maintained at the same time. Admittedly many of these experiments
were crude, but they were conducted simultaneously in comparison with
other isolations of *T. congolense*-like organisms in similar experimental
animals (Tables 2 and 3).

Such trypanosomes of low infectivity to rodents may be common in the
field. As can be seen from Table 4, surveys show that a substantial
proportion of infections is missed when attempting to isolate into
rodents. The infectivity may, of course, depend on the state of the
organism at a particular time, or indeed on the methods used in the
survey; nevertheless, an appreciable number of rodents became infected
but showed only very low grade parasitaemias, indicating a low capability for maintenance in laboratory rodents. There is thus a kind, or
a group of familiar kinds, of *T. congolense*, not uncommon in the field,
that is rarely studied in the laboratory. The lack of virulence to
rodents may suggest that such organisms are unimportant; however, some
of the early work described their pathogenicity to cattle. Until the
pathogenicity is properly examined, it is as well to remember that the
human pathogen *T.b.gambiense* can also fail to infect rodents and when
it does, only low grade parasitaemias may be produced (Godfrey 1977).

Another kind of *T. congolense* described in the literature is that
infecting only pigs, although most stocks infect pigs as well as other
animals. Again, this material is rarely studied because of the difficulty of establishing infections in the laboratory. Confusion arises

Table 2. *T. congolense* infections in dogs (from data by Godfrey 1961)

Type	No. dogs inoculated	Deaths
congolense	2	0
dimorphon	8	8

Table 3. *T. congolense* infections in rats (from data by Godfrey 1961)

Type	No. rats inoculated	No. patent infections	Deaths
congolense	13	5	0
dimorphon	5	5	5

with *T. simiae*, regarded as belonging to the same subgenus as *T. congolense* but reputedly differing in being long, never infecting laboratory rodents and being lethal to pigs. The difference, however, is by no means clear. Péel and Chardome (1954b) and Chardome and Péel (1954) described short trypanosomes that infect only pigs without killing them, and these may resemble the stock of variable pathogenicity reported by Mackenzie and Boyt (1969). Moreover, Roberts (1971) pointed out that a stock of *T. simiae* transmitted by him was virulent only to pigs, did not infect cattle or sheep, but was of a similar size to *T. congolense*.

Many have stated the unreliability of mean length determinations for classifying divisions within trypanosome subgenera (see Godfrey 1977), and this attitude is substantiated by the findings on *T. simiae*. The species may be simply a form of *T. congolense* that is both host-restricted, and pathogenic, to pigs; it may be related to other pig preferring forms that are not pathogenic. Again we shall not appreciate epidemiology fully until the significance and occurrence of the pig adapted kinds are understood. How frequently do they infect other animals? They will not infect rodents, so microscopically subpatent parasitaemias in the field or experimental animals may well be missed; many *Trypanozoon* infections in the field are subpatent.

4.4. Conclusions

Numerous other questions arise concerning the significance of the various kinds of *T. congolense* in nature. Do they occur in particular areas, tsetse or mammals? What is their response to drugs? Can they influence the course of disease when present in a mixture with other strains or species? Mixtures of species occur frequently in areas of high tsetse challenge, and colleagues in Hamburg and ourselves have also shown that different kinds of *Trypanozoon* can occur naturally together in one animal, and persist as a mixed infection (Scott 1981; Schütt and Mehlitz 1981).

Table 4. Isolation of *T. congolense*

Country	Reference	No. and species of host	Total no. infected*	Failed rodent inoculation	Low parasitaemia in rodents	Effective failures to isolate
Nigeria	Godfrey & Killick-Kendrick (1961)	105 cattle	62 (59%) (TF+RI)	10	5	15 (24%)
Nigeria	Killick-Kendrick & Godfrey (1963a)	193 cattle	63 (33%) (TF+RI)	9	5	14 (22%)
Nigeria	Killick-Kendrick & Godfrey (1963b)	35 pigs	29 (83%) (TF+RI)	5	3	8 (28%)
Liberia	Mehlitz (1979)	117 pigs	44 (38%) (TF+HCT+RI)	14	?	14 (32%)
Liberia	Mehlitz (1979)	105 dogs	32 (30%) (TF+HCT+RI)	5	?	5 (16%)
The Gambia	Young (1980)	631 cattle	62 (10%) (HCT+RI)	40	9	49 (79%)

* RI = Rodent inoculation; TF = Thick blood film; HCT = Haematocrit centrifuge technique

How then is the epidemiology of *T. congolense* and its relatives to be investigated? The 'strains' must be recognized accurately, and to do that they must be isolated not just as occasional specimens but on a scale sufficient to validate any characterization method. For all we know, morphological criteria may be adequate, but this remains uncertain until many specimens have been examined. It is likely that the segregation of *T. simiae* by its mean length is an artefact resulting from too few specimens having been studied in detail; the earlier segregation of *T. congolense* from *T. dimorphon* on morphological criteria collapsed when more samples were examined (see Godfrey 1977). It must not be accepted that an identical characteristic among a few stocks means that all *T. congolense*-like organisms are the same in that respect. For instance, DNA buoyant densities were the same, with an unusual component, in the stocks of *T. congolense* examined by Newton and Burnett (1972), but these stocks would be of the kind easily isolated, and any others may well be different.

What prospects are there for isolating and then characterizing a large collection of *T. congolense* stocks? Biochemical or immunological techniques that identify the scarce organisms found in naturally infected hosts may eventually be developed, but at present we must depend on isolation. One method may be the use of immunosuppressed rodents. But such animals, taken to the field in Africa, and maybe kept for many weeks afterwards, run a high risk of dying from intercurrent infections. Another approach may be the use of inbred animals highly susceptible to infection with *T. congolense*. Jennings *et al.* (1978) found certain inbred mice to be more susceptible to disease than others, while Morrison *et al.* (1978) showed that parasitaemias were higher in particular inbred mice; further investigation may find an animal readily infected with low inocula of the various kinds of *T. congolense*. Alternatively, other species of rodents may be useful, rather as the multimammate rat can be used for isolating the recalcitrant kinds of *T. brucei* (Mehlitz 1978). Another approach arises from improvements in methods for *in vitro* multiplication of *T. congolense*, so perhaps one day organisms from any natural infection will be cultured (Gray *et al.* 1981).

Once these major obstacles are overcome, then intrinsic characterization linked with laboratory comparisons of vector transmission, pathogenicity, and host specificity will lead to a much better understanding of the epidemiology of *T. congolense*. In the meanwhile, we must remain aware that the results of laboratory work may not apply to all the kinds existing in the field, albeit sufficiently widespread characterization will adequately describe some of the strains.

Acknowledgement

I acknowledge with thanks partial support from the UNDP/World Bank/WHO Special Programme for Research Training in Tropical Diseases, and the Overseas Development Administration.

44

4.5. References

Bruce, D., Hamerton, A.E., Bateman, H.R., Mackie, F.P. and Bruce, Lady (1911). Sleeping sickness and other diseases of man and animals in Uganda during the years 1908-9-10. No. 30. *Trypanosoma nanum* (Laveran). Reports of the Sleeping Sickness Commission of the Royal Society 2, 164-170.

Chardome, M. and Péel, E. (1954). Étude expérimentale d'une souche appelée *T. congolense* var. *berghei* transmise par *Glossina brevipalpis* du Mosso (Urundi). Annales de la Société belge de Médecine Tropicale 34, 311-320.

Gibson, W.C., Mehlitz, D., Lanham, S.M. and Godfrey, D.G. (1978). The identification of *Trypanosoma brucei gambiense* in Liberian pigs and dogs by isoenzymes and by resistance to human plasma. Tropenmedizin und Parasitologie 29, 335-345.

Gibson, W.C., Marshall, T.F. de C. and Godfrey, D.G. (1980). Numerical analysis of enzyme polymorphism: a new approach to the epidemiology and taxonomy of trypanosomes of the subgenus *Trypanozoon*. Advances in Parasitology 18, 175-246.

Godfrey, D.G. (1961). Types of *Trypanosoma congolense*. II. Differences in the courses of infection. Annals of Tropical Medicine and Parasitology 55, 154-166.

Godfrey, D.G. (1977). Problems in distinguishing between the morphologically similar trypanosomes of mammals. Protozoology 3, 33-49.

Godfrey, D.G. (1979). The zymodemes of trypanosomes. Symposia of the British Society for Parasitology 17, 31-53.

Godfrey, D.G. and Kilgour, V. (1976). Enzyme electrophoresis in characterizing the causative organism of Gambian trypanosomiasis. Transactions of the Royal Society of Tropical Medicine and Hygiene 70, 219-224.

Godfrey, D.G. and Killick-Kendrick, R. (1961). Bovine trypanosomiasis in Nigeria. I - The inoculation of blood into rats as a method of survey in the Donga Valley, Benue Province. Annals of Tropical Medicine and Parasitology 55, 287-295.

Gray, M.A., Cunningham, I., Gardiner, P.R., Taylor, A.M. and Luckins, A.G. (1981). Cultivation of infective forms of *Trypanosoma congolense* from trypanosomes in the proboscis of *Glossina morsitans*. Parasitology 82, 81-95.

Jennings, F.W., Whitelaw, D.D., Holmes, P.H. and Urquhart, G.M. (1978). The susceptibility of strains of mice to infection with *Trypanosoma congolense*. Research in Veterinary Science 25, 399-400.

Killick-Kendrick, R. and Godfrey, D.G. (1963a). Bovine trypanosomiasis in Nigeria. II - The incidence among some migrating cattle with observations on the examination of wet blood preparations as a method of survey. Annals of Tropical Medicine and Parasitology 57, 117-126.

Killick-Kendrick, R. and Godfrey, D.G. (1963b). Observations on a close association between *Glossina tachinoides* and domestic pigs near Nsukka, Eastern Nigeria. I. *Trypanosoma congolense* and *T. brucei* infections in the pigs. Annals of Tropical Medicine and Parasitology 57, 225-231.

Laveran, A. and Mesnil, F. (1912). Trypanosomes et trypanosomiases, edition 2. Masson, Paris.

Leach, T.M. and Roberts, C.J. (1981). Present status of chemotherapy and chemoprophylaxis of animal trypansomiases in the eastern hemisphere. Pharmacology and Therapeutics 13, 91-147.

Mackenzie, P.K.I. and Boyt, W.P. (1969). Notes upon a trypanosome strain resembling *T. congolense* apparently completely adapted to the porcine species. British Veterinary Journal 125, 414-420.

Mehlitz, D. (1978). Untersuchungen zur Empfänglichkeit von *Mastomys natalensis* für *Trypanosoma (Trypanozoon) brucei gambiense*. Tropenmedizin und Parasitologie 29, 101-107.

Mehlitz, D. (1979). Trypanosome infections in domestic animals in Liberia. Tropenmedizin und Parasitologie 30, 212-219.

Mehlitz, D., Zillman, U., Scott, C.M. and Godfrey, D.G. (in press). Epidemiological studies on the animal reservoir of gambian sleeping sickness. Part IV. Characterization of *Trypanozoon* stocks by isoenzymes and sensitivity to human serum. Tropenmedizin und Parasitologie.

Miles, M.A., Povoa, M.M., De Souza, A.A., Lainson, R., Shaw, J.J. and Ketteridge, D.S. (1981). Chagas' disease in the Amazon Basin: II. The distribution of *Trypanosoma cruzi* zymodemes 1 and 3 in Pará State, north Brazil. Transactions of the Royal Society of Tropical Medicine and Hygiene 75, 667-674.

Morrison, W.I., Roelants, G.E., Mayor-Withey, K.S. and Murray, M. (1978). Susceptibility of inbred strains of mice to *Trypanosoma congolense*: correlation with changes in spleen lymphocyte populations. Clinical and Experimental Immunology 32, 25-40.

Newton, B.A. and Burnett, J.K. (1972). DNA of Kinetoplastidae: a comparative study, in Comparative Biochemistry of Parasites (edited by H. Van den Bossche), pp. 185-198. Academic Press, London.

Péel, E. and Chardome, M. (1954a). Étude expérimentale d'une souche considérée comme *T. congolense* Broden 1904 et transmise par *Glossina brevipalpis* du Mosso (Urundi). Annales de la Société Belge de Médecine Tropicale 34, 297-302.

Péel, E. and Chardome, M. (1954b). Étude expérimentale d'une souche appelée *T. congolense* var. *urundiense* transmise par *Glossina brevipalpis* du Mosso (Urundi). Annales de la Société Belge de Médecine Tropicale 34, 303-310.

Roberts, C.J. (1971). The lack of infectivity to cattle of a strain of *Trypanosoma simiae* transmitted by *Glossina morsitans* and *G. tachinoides*. Annals of Tropical Medicine and Parasitology 65, 319-326.

Schütt, I.D. and Mehlitz, D. (1981). On the persistence of human serum resistance and isoenzyme patterns of *Trypanozoon* clones in experimentally infected pigs. Acta Tropica <u>38</u>, 367-373.

Scott, C.M. (1981). Mixed populations of *Trypanosoma brucei* in a naturally infected pig. Tropenmedizin und Parasitologie <u>32</u>, 221-222.

Sneath, P.H.A. and Sokal, R.R. (1973). Numerical taxonomy. Freeman, San Francisco.

Young, C.J. (1980). Zymodemes of *Trypanosoma congolense* and a preliminary assessment of their epidemiological significance. Ph. D. thesis, University of London.

CHAPTER 5
Chemotherapy of Chagas's Disease

W.E. Gutteridge

Biological Laboratory,
University of Kent,
Canterbury, Kent, CT2 7NU.

(Present address:
Wellcome Research Laboratories,
Langley Court, Beckenham,
Kent, BR3 3BS.)

5.1. Introduction

   Chagas's disease remains a major health problem in Latin America.
According to the usually quoted figures, about 35 million people live
in areas where it is endemic and at least 12 million are actually
infected (Brener 1979; Gutteridge 1980). The disease presents two
problems as far as chemotherapy is concerned. First, there is a need
to treat patients who have become naturally infected with *Trypanosoma
cruzi* as a result of being bitten by an infected triatomid bug.
Second, there is the need to prevent transmission of the disease from
an infected donor to a non-infected recipient during blood transfusion.
The solutions required for these two problems are quite distinct and
so I will deal with them separately.

5.2. Drugs for treatment

   The characteristic feature of *T. cruzi*, the causative agent of
Chagas's disease, is that the main replicative form in the mammal, the
amastigote, develops intracellularly. Work, particularly in my own
laboratory, over a number of years suggests that there is no redund-
ancy of major biochemical pathways as a result of this intracellular
development (see Gutteridge and Rogerson 1979 for review), so that
there is no parallel here with the problems associated with anti-viral
chemotherapy. Clearly, however, there is in Chagas's disease an
additional pharmacological barrier to be overcome, in getting drug to
the parasite, that does not occur in, for example, the African trypanosomiases. In addition, any mechanism of selective toxicity cannot
rely, as many African trypanosomicides appear to do, on differential
permeability of drug between host and parasite cells (see Gutteridge

Table 1. Current status of compounds tested clinically for activity
   in Chagas's disease (reproduced with permission from Gutteridge
   1980, slightly modified).

Date synthesised	Class	Example	Current status
1937	Bisquinaldines	Bayer 7602 Ac	Abandoned
1938	Arsenobenzenes	Spirotrypan	Abandoned
1946	Phenanthridines	Carbidium	Abandoned
1949	8-Aminoquinolines	Primaquine	Abandoned
1974		Moxipraquine	Abandoned
1952	5-Nitrofurans	Nitrofurazone	Abandoned
1972		Nifurtimox	Released
1961	5-Nitroimidazoles	Metronidazole	Abandoned
1979		MK 436	Experimental tests
1979		Fexinidazole	Experimental tests
1966	5-Nitrothiazoles	Niridazole	Abandoned
1968	2-Nitroimidazoles	-	Abandoned
1974		Benznidazole	Released

and Coombs 1977 for review). Not surprisingly, therefore, only a
limited number of drugs has been found to be active in experimental
Chagas's disease and only eight classes of these have proceeded to
clinical trials (Gutteridge 1980).

The current state of development of these eight classes is shown in
Table 1. No new class has been discovered since 1968; only three
series are at present under investigation - the 5-nitrofurans, the
5-nitroimidazoles and 2-nitroimidazoles, all of which are nitrohetero-
cycles; and only two drugs are on the market, Nifurtimox (synonyms:
Bayer 2502, Lampit; structure: Figure 1) which was introduced in 1976
(Bock *et al*. 1972) and Benznidazole (synonyms:Ro 7-1051, Radanil;
structure: Figure 2) which was released in late 1978 (Richle 1974).

There has been considerable controversy over the years, both orally
and in the literature, about the overall efficacy of these two drugs.
The dust, however, has now settled enough for four main points of
agreement to have emerged. First, there is apparently little to
choose between the efficacy and toxicity of Nifurtimox and Benznidazole.
Second, both drugs are valuable in preventing death as a result of
acute infection with *T. cruzi*. Third, neither drug is well tolerated
by patients over the periods of time (60-120 days) normally used in
attempts to cure chronic cases. Patients suffer nausea, loss of weight

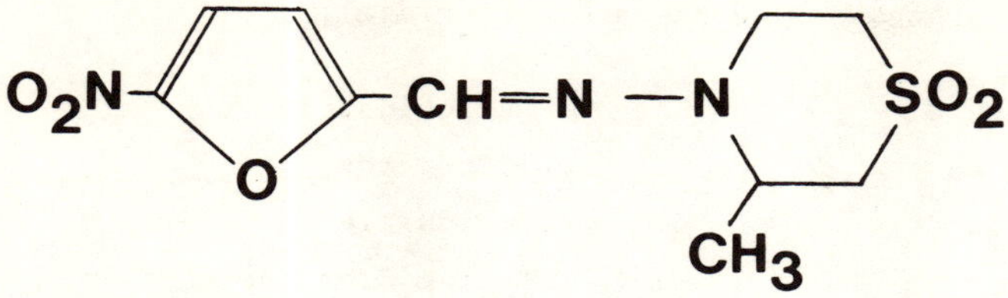

Figure 1. Nifurtimox.

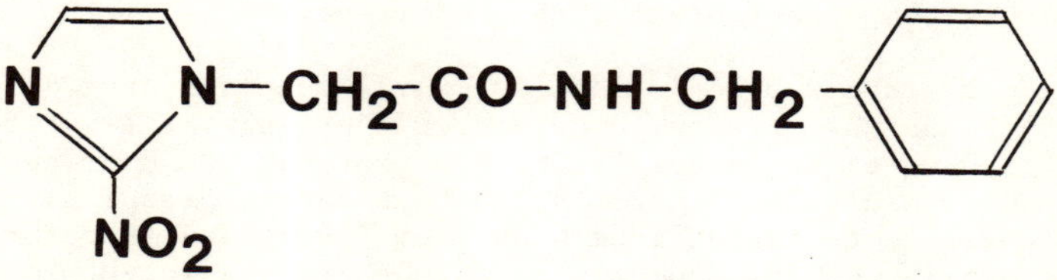

Figure 2. Benznidazole.

and general malaise and depression such that few complete the full treatment period. Fourth, there is considerable variation in the cure rates for chronic infections in different parts of Latin America. As a general rule, cure rates are high in the south of the continent and decrease as one goes north (Cerisola 1977), to such an extent that in the northern parts of Brazil, most clinicians apparently will use the drugs for acute cases only. This variation in efficacy apparently relates to variation in the sensitivity of different strains of *T. cruzi* to these drugs (see Cover and Gutteridge 1981 for review). Just how far such variation will be a problem in the future remains to be seen; Nifurtimox and Benznidazole are being used at their maximum tolerated doses so that there is no possibility of even small increases in dosages.

Overall, it is clear that there are deficiencies in existing drugs used for the treatment of chronic cases of Chagas's disease. A number of approaches is being tried in attempts to overcome this problem. One, which was tried in my own laboratory a number of years ago, was to look for synergism among existing compounds experimentally active (Dignasse, Squance and Gutteridge, unpublished observations). The work, done independently in duplicate employed the non-pathogen, *Trypanosoma dionisii, in vitro* as test system (see Gaborak *et al.* 1977 for validation of its use). Initial experiments involved the determination of the concentrations of the drugs listed in Table 2 which caused

Table 2. Drugs tested *in vitro* in all permutations of two for synergistic activity against *Trypanosoma dionisii* (unpublished results of Dignasse, Squance and Gutteridge).

Amphotericin B	Metronidazole
Bayer 7602 Ac	Nifurtimox
Benznidazole	Niridazole
Cordycepin	Pentamidine isethionate
Ethidium bromide	Spirotrypan
Merck 436	

a 10-20% decrease in the rate of growth of the organism. The drugs were then tested at these concentrations in all permutations of two. In no case was the effect greater than additive.

Another approach has been to look for novel means of drug delivery, either with liposomes or with lysosomotropic drugs. At least two laboratories have tried encapsulating 5-nitrofuran and 8-aminoquinolines in liposomes. Results were negative in both cases, presumably because it is not possible to target them away from liver, and therefore have never been published. Lysosomotropic chemotherapy using ethidium bromide-DNA complexes has also been attempted, with what were thought initially to be encouraging results (Trouet *et al*. 1976). It is now generally accepted, however, that the prolongation of life observed in the experimental animals was the result of drug depot effects.

The main approach to overcoming the current inadequacies of the chemotherapy of Chagas's disease has been to attempt new drug development. This is being done both empirically and rationally. Empirical work has led to the identification of two new drugs active in experimental Chagas's disease. Both are 5-nitroimidazoles and both were announced in 1979. MK 436 (structure:Figure 3) has been shown to be active against B, Y and C strains of *T. cruzi* in both mice and dogs (Miller *et al*. 1979a and b; Malanga *et al*. 1981). Fexinidazole (synonym:HOE 239; structure:Figure 4) cleared not only parasitaemia, but also pseudocysts from the myocardium (Raether and Deutschlander 1979). It is still too early for results to have emerged from possible clinical trials but there is nothing in the experimental data so far to suggest that either compound is markedly more active than Nifurtimox or Benznidazole.

The rational approach has concentrated on studying the comparative biochemistry of host and parasite and the mechanism of action of drugs active *in vitro* against *T. cruzi*. As I discussed in a recent review (Gutteridge 1980) and as Table 3 shows, it has been very successful in identifying targets potentially susceptible to chemotherapeutic attack, but so far, because it is not normally possible to involve teams of chemists in the work, it has been less successful in producing

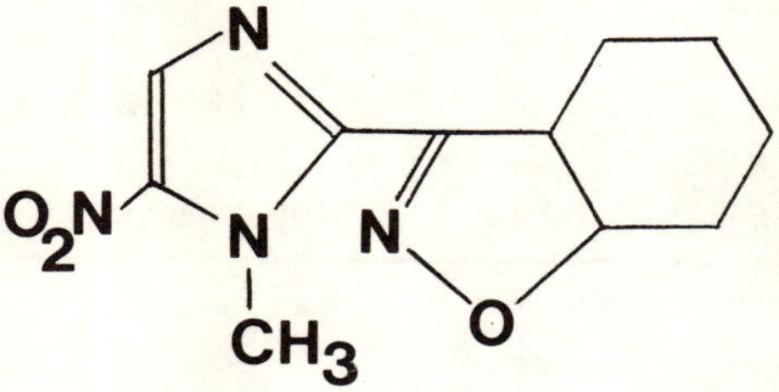

Figure 3.   MK 436.

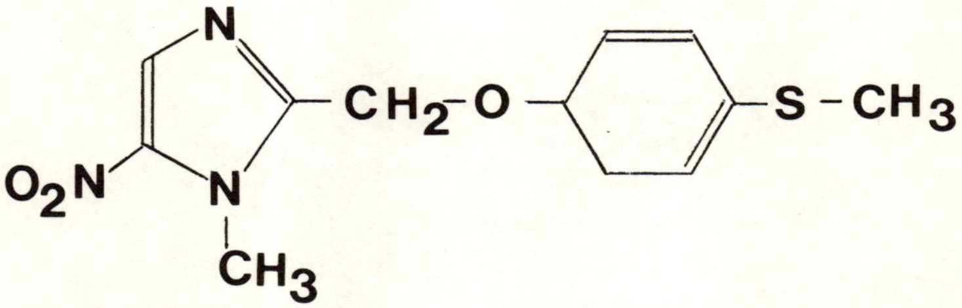

Figure 4.   Fexinidazole.

compounds with activity *in vivo*. One example here, about which we have not perhaps heard the last, is allopurinol (structure:Figure 5) which has been in clinical use for the treatment of gout for a number of years. Marr and his co-workers (1978) showed that *T. cruzi* metabolizes the compound differently to man. The nucleotide product of this metabolism is active against the trypanosome *in vitro*, though not, it now appears, against nucleic acid and protein synthesis as reported originally, but rather against the inter-conversion of purines. Unfortunately, with one notable exception (Avila and Avila 1981), no one can find activity experimentally *in vivo*, probably because the drug is metabolized and/or excreted too rapidly by the host. There are unconfirmed rumours, however, that despite this, it is being tried clinically in Latin America.

I am sorry, therefore, to have to conclude this part of my paper with the message that not only is the current chemotherapy for the treatment of Chagas's disease inadequate, but that this is likely to remain the situation for a number of years.

Table 3. Targets with possible chemotherapeutic potential in
Trypanosoma cruzi (reproduced with permission from Gutteridge 1980,
slightly modified).

Target metabolic area	Possible target	Target identified by study of:	
		Comparative biochemistry	Mode of action of drugs
Carbohydrate & energy	Energy reserves	+	
	Unusual substrates	+	
	Glycosome	+	
	Rapid flow of PP shunt	+	
	Cytochrome o	+	
	Cytochrome c$_{558}$	+	
	Ubiquinones		+
	Fumarate reductase	+	
	NADH oxidase	+	
	α-Glycerophosphate oxidation	+	
	Glutamate dehydrogenase	+	
Nucleic acids	DNA		+
	Kinetoplast DNA		+
	Dihydrofolate reductase	+	+
	Thymidylate synthase	+	
	Dihydroorotate hydroxylase	+	
	Pyrazolopyrimidine metabolism		+
	DNA & RNA polymerases		+
	Nucleic acid synthesis		+
Protein and lipid	Amino acid transport	+	
	Sterols	+	+
	Fatty acid synthesis from threonine	+	
General	Absence of catalase	+	+

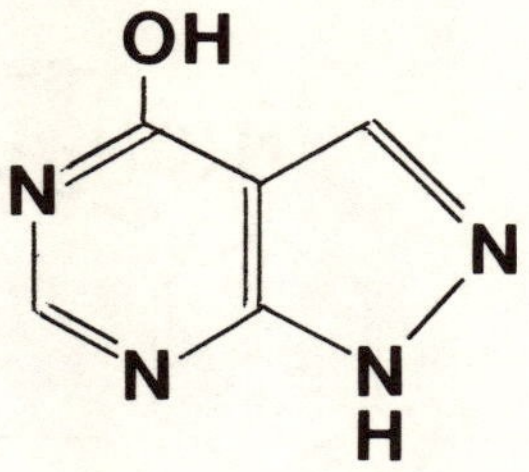

Figure 5. Allopurinol.

5.3. Drugs to prevent transmission during blood transfusion

The problem here is that if blood from a donor suffering from
Chagas's disease is not treated to kill any trypomastigotes which
it may contain, the infection will probably be transmitted to the
recipient of that blood. The incidence of *T. cruzi* infection in blood
banks in Latin America ranges from 1.3-28%, depending on the location
investigated; evidence for transmission of the disease was found in
13-19% of patients who received blood from Chagasic donors (Rassi and
De Rezende 1976). In theory, this problem is simpler than that posed
by infected patients, since one is dealing only with extracellular
trypomastigote forms of the parasite and therefore the pharmacological
problems are less acute.

The danger of transmission is overcome at present by adding gentian
violet (Figure 6) to the blood and storing it at 4°C for at least 24 h
(Nussensweig *et al.* 1953). This ensures that the trypomastigotes are
lysed and hence rendered non-infective. There are three problems with
this solution. First, the safety of using gentian violet in this way
has never been assessed. Second, the drug is used at such a high
concentration ($\sim$1mM) that it colours the blood bright purple, so that
it is not always acceptable to patients. Third, the protocol for its
use has to be followed exactly, particularly with respect to the time
and temperature of storage, which is not always possible in all parts of
Latin America. Clearly, therefore, there is the need for a replacement for gentian violet. The problem is that only rarely has such a
replacement been sought directly. The goal of most screening programmes
against *T. cruzi* has been a drug for treatment. Only when this has
been discovered is it tested for trypanosomicidal activity against
infected whole blood stored *in vitro* at 4°C. This is a pity, because
as I indicated earlier, the pharmacological problems which render the
chemotherapy of Chagas's disease so difficult are not a problem here
and testing can be done readily *in vitro*.

This last point is best illustrated by the primary screening system
that we have developed recently in Canterbury (Cover and Gutteridge
in press). A drop of mouse blood infected with *T. cruzi* is mixed with
a similarly sized drop of drug solution, loaded into a Microslide tube

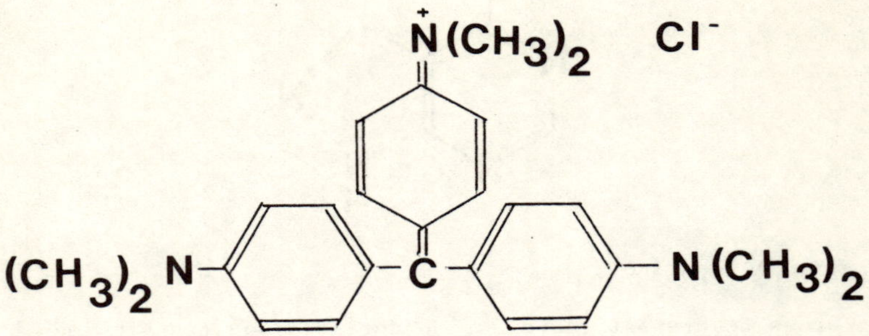

Figure 6. Gentian violet.

and incubated overnight in a wet-box at 4°C before being assessed for
the number of trypomastigotes by direct microscopic examination. Some
of the results obtained during the development of this system are
shown in Table 4. Note particularly the efficacy of gentian violet,
the absence of effect of Nifurtimox and Benznidazole (the two drugs
used in the treatment of Chagas's disease which are trypanosomicidal at
37°C), and the activity of the polyene antibiotic, amphotericin B,
and the arsenical, spirotrypan; both of the latter are already known
to be active in this respect, though unfortunately they are too toxic
for clinical use (Cruz *et al*. 1980; Mieth and Seidenath 1967).

We are hoping to use this system to screen a large number of compounds, concentrating initially on those that already have a product
licence and can therefore be used with a minimum of safety testing.

5.4. Conclusions

The emphasis of the seminar was on current inadequacies. As far as
Chagas's disease is concerned, there are two. First, we still need
a drug well tolerated by patients which will in a single or small
number of doses cure patients with chronic Chagas's disease in all
parts of Latin America. Second, we need a stable colourless (or red!)
compound which when added to blood intended for use in transfusion
will, within minutes, destroy all the trypomastigotes present, whether
the blood is stored at 4° or room temperature.

Table 4. Effects of drugs on trypomastigotes of *T. cruzi in vitro* (data by Cover and Gutteridge, in press).

Drug (final concentration 0.5 mM)	Trypomastigotes*
Control	+
Gentian violet	−
Crystal violet	−
Amphotericin B	−
Spirotrypan	−
Nifurtimox	+
Nitrofurazone	+
SQ18506	+
Benznidazole	+
Ethidium bromide	+
Bayer 7602 Ac	+
Allopurinol	+
Hydrogen peroxide	+

* +, same number present as in control preparation
  −, all organisms lysed

Acknowledgements

   The author's work referred to in this paper was financed by the Overseas Development Ministry and the Medical Research Council, London and the World Health Organization, Geneva.

5.5. References

Avila, J.L. and Avila, A. (1981). *Trypanosoma cruzi*: allopurinol in the treatment of mice with experimental acute Chagas' disease. Experimental Parasitology 51, 204-208.

Bock, M., Haberkorn, A., Herlinger, H., Mayer, K.H. and Petersen, S. (1972). The structure-activity relationship of 4-(5[1]-nitrofurfurylidene-amino)-tetrahydro-4H-1,4-thiazine-1,1-dioxides against *Trypanosoma cruzi*. Arzneimittel Forschung 22, 1564-1569.

56

Brener, Z. (1979). Present status of chemotherapy and chemoprophylaxis of human trypanosomiasis in the Western hemisphere. Pharmacology and Therapeutics 7, 71-90.

Cerisola, J.A. (1977). Chemotherapy of Chagas' infection in man, in Chagas' Disease, pp. 35-47. Pan American Health Organization, Washington D.C. (Scientific Publication number 347.)

Cover, B. and Gutteridge, W.E. (1981). Comparison of drug sensitivities of three strains of *Trypanosoma cruzi* in inbred A/JAX mice. Transactions of the Royal Society of Tropical Medicine and Hygiene 75, 274-281.

Cover, B. and Gutteridge, W.E. (in press). A primary screen for drugs to prevent transmission of Chagas' disease during blood transfusion. Transactions of the Royal Society of Tropical Medicine and Hygiene.

Cruz, F.S., Marr, J.J. and Berens, R.L. (1980). Prevention of transfusion-induced Chagas' disease by amphotericin B. American Journal of Tropical Medicine and Hygiene 29, 761-765.

Gaborak, M., Darling J.L. and Gutteridge, W.E. (1977). *Trypanosoma cruzi* and *Trypanosoma dionisii*: comparative drug sensitivities of culture forms. Nature 268, 339-340.

Gutteridge, W.E. (1980). Prospects for chemotherapy of Chagas' disease, in The Host-Invader Interplay (edited by H. Van den Bossche), pp. 583-594. Elsevier/North Holland Biomedical Press, Amsterdam.

Gutteridge, W.E. and Coombs, G.H. (1977). Biochemistry of Parasitic Protozoa. Macmillan, London.

Gutteridge, W.E. and Rogerson, G.W. (1979). Biochemical aspects of the biology of *Trypanosoma cruzi*, in Biology of the Kinetoplastida (edited by W.H.R. Lumsden and D.A. Evans), pp. 619-652. Academic Press, London, New York and San Francisco.

Malanga, C.M., Conroy, J. and Cuckler, A.C. (1981). Therapeutic efficacy of several nitroimidazoles for experimental *Trypanosoma cruzi* infections in mice. Journal of Parasitology 67, 35-40.

Marr, J.J., Berens, R.L. and Nelson, D.J. (1978). Antitrypanosomal effect of allopurinol: conversion in vivo to aminopyrazolopyrimidine nucleotides by *Trypanosoma cruzi*. Science 201, 1018-1020.

Mieth, H. and Seidenath, H. (1967). Chemotherapeutische Untersuchungen an *Trypanosoma cruzi* in der Gewebekultur. Zeitschrift für Tropenmedizin und Parasitologie 18, 53-60.

Miller, B.M., Malanga, C.M., Taylor, J. and Conroy, J. (1979a). Efficacy of MK 436, a substituted 5-nitroimidazole, against *Trypanosoma cruzi* in mice. Congresso Internacional Sobre Doença de Chagas, Rio de Janeiro, p. 140.

Miller, B.M., Malanga, C.M. and Conroy, J. (1979b). Efficacy of MK 436, a substituted 5-nitroimidazole, against *Trypanosoma cruzi* in dogs. Congresso Internacional Sobre Doença de Chagas, Rio de Janeiro, p. 141.

Nussenweig, V., Biancalana, A., Amato Neta, V., Sonntag, R., Freitas, J.L.P. and Kloetzel, J. (1953). Acao da violeta de genciana sobre o *T. cruzi* in vitro: sua importancia na esterilizacao do sangue destinado a transfusao. Revista Paulista de Medicina 42, 57-58.

Raether, W. and Deutschlander, N. (1979). HOE 239 (Fexinidazole), a 5-nitroimidazole highly potent against *Trypanosoma cruzi* in NMRI mice. Congresso Internacional Sobre Doenca de Chagas, Rio de Janeiro, p. 142.

Rassi, A. and De Rezende, J.M. (1976). Prevention of transmission of *T. cruzi* by blood transfusion, in American Trypanosomiasis Research, pp. 273-278. Pan American Health Organization, Washington, D.C. (Scientific Publication number 318.)

Richle, R. (1974). Chemotherapy of experimental acute Chagas' disease in mice: parasitological cure by Ro 7-1051. Proceedings of the Third International Congress of Parasitology, München 3, 1296-1297.

Trouet, A., Jadin, J.-M. and Van Hoof, F. (1976). Lysosomotropic chemotherapy in protozoal diseases, in Biochemistry of Parasites and Host-Parasite Relationships (edited by H. Van den Bossche), pp. 519-522. Elsevier/North Holland Biomedical Press, Amsterdam.

CHAPTER 6
Chemotherapy Against Animal Trypanosomiasis

P.H. Holmes

University of Glasgow Veterinary School,
Bearsden Road,
Glasgow, G61 1QH

and

J.M. Scott

Overseas Development Administration,
Eland House, Stag Place,
London, SW1E 5DH.

6.1. Introduction

Although animal trypanosomiasis is a world-wide problem in tropical countries, the major veterinary and economic impact of the disease is undoubtedly in African cattle. For this reason our paper is largely concerned with current problems in the treatment of African bovine trypanosomiasis, although many aspects are pertinent to situations other than in Africa.

The essential question posed was 'Why are current methods of chemotherapy inadequate?'. In answer, we suggest that in many situations the methods are not as inadequate as is commonly supposed but it is their application which is so often unsatisfactory.

However, let us first briefly consider some of the better known pharmacological problems associated with chemotherapy. More detailed accounts of these problems have been presented in extensive reviews by Whiteside (1962), Williamson (1970) and Rüchel (1975).

6.2. Pharmacological problems

6.2.1. Range of available drugs

One of the widely recognized problems associated with chemotherapy against animal trypanosomiasis is that the number of effective drugs is extremely limited and no new drug has been marketed since the early

1960s. Indeed the situation has deteriorated because antrycide, which was in widespread use for many years, ceased to be manufactured in 1976. Thus there are now only four drugs in use in Africa, namely Ethidium (Homidium bromide), Prothidium (Pyrithidium bromide), Samorin (Isometamidium chloride) and Berenil (Diminazene aceturate). Of these, Samorin and Berenil are the most widely used and most readily available.

6.2.2. Drug resistance

The other well known problem in the field is that of drug resistance. There is substantial evidence from many areas of Africa that drug resistant strains of trypanosomes are widespread. Furthermore, there is a considerable degree of cross-resistance between the commonly available drugs (see review by Williamson 1970). However, there are several important factors which may reduce the veterinary impact of this problem in the field. First, cross-resistance between the two most commonly used drugs, Samorin and Berenil, is very rarely observed in the field. Secondly, resistance to Berenil, although reported, occurs relatively infrequently. Thirdly, there is some evidence from the field that drug resistant strains may often be of comparatively low pathogenicity (Goble *et al.* 1959; Stephen 1962), but this requires confirmation.

It is also important to define the various forms of drug resistance which have been described. While drug resistance may be relatively straightforward, in the sense of a very limited or ineffectual res-ponse of parasitaemia to treatment, there are other situations in which the term 'drug resistance' requires qualification. For example, resistance may be observed at only relatively low levels of drug dosage. It is also possible that a form of relapse may occur after drug therapy, which is directly related to the interval of time between infection and treatment. Such a phenomenon has been reported in mice by Jennings *et al.* (1977), who showed that there was a correlation between duration of infection with *Trypanosoma brucei* and the efficacy of chemotherapy. Thus mice treated soon (3 days) after infection were permanently cured, using a variety of drugs. However, if treatment was delayed until 14-21 days after infection, none of the available trypanosomicidal drugs produced a permanent cure, even if used at dose rates far in excess of those recommended. Treatment 14-21 days after infection was followed by a period without parasitaemia, but eventually (up to 7 months later) trypanosomes reappeared in the blood. During the apara-sitaemic period the only organ in the body of the treated mouse capable of transferring infection to an uninfected recipient was the brain (Jennings *et al.* 1979). Current evidence supports the view that this was because insufficient amounts of drug passed the blood-brain barr-iers to eliminate the infection.

Whether or not this form of relapsing infection following chemotherapy occurs in cattle has yet to be determined. However, it is of interest that there are three reports from Nigeria (MacLennan and Na'isa 1970; MacLennan 1971; Gray and Roberts 1971) describing infections of *T. vivax* and *T. congolense* which generally relapsed 10 to 40 days after chemo-

Table 1. Toxic effects of drugs in current use against animal trypanosomiasis.

Drug	Dose mg/kg (intramuscular)	Toxic effects
Ethidium Prothidium Samorin	0.5 - 2	Local tissue damage common in cattle. Toxic to camels.
Berenil	3.5 - 7	Usually negligible in cattle. Abscess formation in horses. Often fatal in camels and dogs.

therapy.

6.2.3. Drug toxicity

It is well recognized that many drugs are limited in their use because of the severe toxic reactions they induce in a number of domestic
species (Table 1). Furthermore, even drugs that are relatively safe
to use in terms of mortality often cause marked tissue reactions at
the site of injection. This is particularly true of Prothidium and
Samorin and, to prevent lameness and damage to the hindquarters of
cattle, it is usually recommended that these drugs are injected into
the neck muscles. Though this practice is generally acceptable, it
may cause special problems in draught oxen.

A further problem which will probably receive increasing attention
is that of drug residues in food animals.

6.2.4. Duration of chemoprophylaxis

The duration of chemoprophylaxis is a very important aspect of chemotherapy (Table 2). The period of protection may vary considerably for
several reasons, some of which are not yet fully understood.

One interesting problem is the relationship between prophylaxis and
drug excretion. Several years ago it was reported that curative drugs
such as Berenil may have prophylactic effects of several weeks' duration (Van Hoeve and Cunningham 1964), yet earlier studies had suggested
that Berenil was very rapidly excreted and therefore had no prophylactic
effect (Bauer 1958). A similar type of discrepancy has been reported
from studies on the pharmacokinetics of Ethidium bromide. In the
field, prophylactic activity of this compound has been claimed to
extend over many weeks. However, recent laboratory studies with
[14]C-labelled Ethidium bromide have shown that the drug is very rapidly
excreted, over 93% being eliminated with 96 hours (Gilbert and Newton
in press). There is some evidence to suggest that the explanation may be
that the immune response of the host contributes significantly to the

62

Table 2. Duration of prophylaxis of drugs in current use against
animal trypanosomiasis.

Drug	Dose mg/kg (intramuscular)	Duration
Ethidium	1	6 weeks
Prothidium	2	6 months
Samorin	1-2	4 months
Berenil	7	3 weeks

prophylactic effects observed in treated animals (Goodwin and Tierney 1977; Gilbert and Newton in press).

A related phenomenon is the observation that the duration of chemo-prophylaxis may be reduced in areas of high tsetse challenge (White-side 1962). It has been suggested that one possible reason may be that the drug is taken up by invading trypanosomes, thus reducing the duration of prophylaxis (Davey 1957). It is therefore of interest that in the recent studies with ^{14}C-Ethidium bromide (Gilbert *et al*. 1979), no difference in drug distribution or excretion rate was observed between normal and *T. congolense* infected calves, although in the latter animals 80% of the radioactivity was bound to trypano-somes 1 hour after injection. Hence it appears unlikely that reduced prophylaxis in areas of high challenge is associated with increased drug excretion. However it is possible that the host's immune response, which may be making a significant contribution to prophylaxis in drug treated animals, is impaired in animals under heavy challenge. Immunosuppression in the form of reduced antibody titres to vaccine antigens has been demonstrated in both experimental and natural tryp-anosome infections of cattle (Holmes *et al*. 1974; Scott *et al*. 1977). Furthermore, the level of immunosuppression is apparently related to the level of parasitaemia (Whitelaw *et al*. 1979). Thus it is possible that trypanosome-induced immunosuppression may impair the host's protective immune response and this may be manifested as reduced prophylaxis in areas of high challenge.

Clearly the interrelationship between chemotherapy and immune res-ponse requires further study since it has important practical implic-ations both in conventional chemotherapy programmes and also in the development of drug-assisted acquired trypanotolerance (see below, section 6.4).

6.3. Logistical and financial problems

It is unfortunate that, in general, the countries most severely affected by animal trypanosomiasis are also those which have the low-est gross national product and the poorest ratio of veterinarians to livestock unit (Braend 1979). It is therefore critical that trypano-somiasis control must be fully integrated with agricultural programmes

and be part of realistic land development schemes. Expensive projects
for the treatment of livestock and/or eradication of tsetse flies are
justified only if they allow utilization of unused resources, which
is in the best interest of the general development of the country.
The economics of trypanosomiasis and tsetse control are governed more
by the possible benefits to agriculture than by the cost of control
schemes (Jahnke 1974). Nevertheless at the present time logistical
and financial problems are a major restraint on the effective application of chemotherapy in the field. They include a number of inter-
related factors, discussed in the next sections.

6.3.1. Affected land area

A major difficulty associated with all control measures against
trypanosomiasis is the scale of the problem. Firstly, the area is
vast, *i.e.* 10 million km^2. Secondly, most affected areas are poorly
developed because of the trypanosomiasis and therefore lacking in
essential services. Thirdly, endemic areas are rarely circumscribed
and therefore, because of constant encroachment, rapid elimination of
trypanosomiasis by chemotherapy and/or tsetse control is rarely
feasible.

6.3.2. Communications and facilities

Many control schemes are severely hampered by the general lack of
all-weather road systems; scarcities of vehicles and fuel; absence of
laboratory services for diagnostic purposes; inadequate cattle handling
facilities and erratic supplies of imported drugs, syringes, needles,
etc.

6.3.3. Personnel

All efficient control schemes require the services of permanent
staff who are well trained and highly motivated. Unfortunately, such
personnel are rarely available in adequate numbers.

6.3.4. Education

Good co-operation and enthusiasm by livestock owners and government
officers is vital and must be encouraged by education projects and
training schemes. The cost effectiveness of different control measures
including chemotherapy must be fully evaluated and demonstrated.

6.3.5. Finance

The cost of drugs and the infrastructure required for their distribution and use is considerable and frequently beyond the means of
small farmers. Therefore aid programmes and government support are
essential but, unfortunately, often lacking due to other priorities.

One other common financial difficulty is that of comparing the
relative cost benefits of chemotherapy programmes with tsetse control.

Unfortunately, few detailed cost evaluations have been published but one valuable source of reference is the work of Jahnke (1974). He showed that where the costs of tsetse control are high, the protection of cattle by drugs is preferable unless the incidence of trypanosomiasis and the stock carrying capacity are high. In other words, in high potential land with a high incidence of trypanosomiasis, tsetse control constitutes the method of choice. The lower the stock carrying capacity and the lower the incidence of trypanosomiasis, the more preferable it becomes to protect cattle by drugs instead of controlling tsetse.

6.3.6. Political structure

In the recent past, political instability has been a major factor in disrupting control schemes. As a result, trypanosomiasis has frequently re-emerged as a serious problem in areas in which it was previously controlled.

6.4. Successful chemotherapy schemes

Despite the pharmacological problems described in section 6.2, success can be achieved using currently available drugs if the difficulties outlined in section 6.3 are minimised. In other words, in our opinion logistical and financial problems are a greater barrier than pharmacological problems in implementing successful chemotherapy programmes. Some examples will be given to illustrate the level of success which may be achieved.

The first relates to a ranching scheme in Tanzania. For twenty years Samorin and Berenil have been used on the Mkwaja Ranch in northern Tanzania to control trypanosomiasis in some 15 000 cattle. The cattle are often under heavy challenge from *Glossina morsitans* and ranching has been possible only by the use of chemotherapy. Details of the ranch and its ecology have been described by Ford and Blaser (1971). In the mid-1970's two experiments were conducted with a view to rationalizing the use of Samorin and Berenil in the herd (Blaser *et al*. 1979). In the first experiment 100 calves were selected after weaning and divided into three groups: group A (40 calves) received treatment with Samorin; group B (40 calves) received Berenil; and the remaining 20 calves, group C, were untreated controls. In the two treated groups (A and B), the normal ranch procedure of delaying treatment until about 10% of a particular herd developed detectable parasitaemia was adopted. All three groups were then monitored for 30 months. At the end of this time 90% of the untreated controls had died, whilst in the treated animals the mortality rate was 17.5% and 45% for groups A and B respectively. Furthermore the body weight gains were higher in the treated groups A and B than in group C. Although the cause of death was not recorded for each individual animal, it was clear that trypanosomiasis was a major cause of mortality since the only difference in treatment between the groups was in their chemoprophylaxis.

In the second experiment four groups of twenty calves were selected

and treatments began between four and six weeks of age. Groups D and
E were given Samorin and Berenil respectively at intervals of two
months regardless of the detection of parasitaemias. Group F received
Berenil at the time at which the remainder of the herd was treated on
the basis of 10% level of detectable parasitaemia, and group G
remained untreated throughout the 15 month experiment. At the end of
the study the mortality rates in groups D,E,F and G were 5%, 35%, 20%
and 45% respectively. In addition the body weight gains in the Samorin
treated group (D) were considerably higher than in the other groups.

The results of these studies seem to demonstrate the efficient level
of protection offered by chemoprophylaxis under ranching conditions
in Africa. Furthermore, it is particularly noteworthy that drug
resistance has not emerged as a major problem on the ranch despite
reliance on chemotherapy for twenty years.

The second example is from western Ethiopia and involves the introduction and maintenance of 450 work oxen on a settlement scheme in an
area of high tsetse challenge by the strategic use of trypanosomicidal
drugs (Bourn and Scott 1978). Before 1970 the Angar-Gutin valley was
largely uninhabited, primarily because the dense infestation of tsetse
made the keeping of domestic stock impossible. In 1970 the area was
selected for settlement in a carefully supervised project to resettle
gradually displaced peasants from the Ethiopian Highlands. The aim
of the project was to develop an integrated rural society incorporating
sound land use principles with maize, cotton and peppers as the main
products. The project management believed that it would not be appropriate to introduce mechanization to peasant farmers but instead
that they should rely on work oxen which are widely used in highland
Ethiopia. The first 40 oxen were introduced in 1972 and then gradually
increased in numbers each year as more peasants joined the settlement
and additional land was cleared. Initially the oxen were given block
treatment with Berenil whenever signs of trypanosomiasis appeared in
several of them; on average this was necessary every 28 days. Subsequent attempts to rely solely on a prophylactic drug, Samorin, were
not successful because of the development of drug-resistant strains
of *T. congolense*. For the remaining 3 years of the study Samorin and
Berenil were used alternatively, generally in clinically affected
individuals only and, despite the percentage of oxen with positive
blood films remaining around 50-69%, the number of animals requiring
therapy dropped to approximately 20% per month. It should be stressed
that trypanosomiasis control in the oxen was essentially based on an
empirical approach to the problem with different tactics developed to
cope with changing situations. As a result of this method of control,
fewer than 20 oxen died as a direct result of trypanosomiasis during
the 5 year period 1972-77, the vast majority of animals remaining in
productive work.

This study clearly demonstrated that with careful management, good
veterinary supervision and the judicious use of drugs, a very acceptable level of trypanosomiasis control can be achieved in areas of
high tsetse challenge using available methods, essentially because of

the animals's ability to develop an adequate level of non-sterile
immunity with the assistance of chemotherapy.

Bevan (1928) was apparently the first to suggest that 'vaccination'
or 'tolerance' might be produced in cattle by giving a trypanosomicidal
drug after infection with a laboratory-passaged strain of *T. congolense*.
However, it was a series of experiments in East Africa by Wilson and
colleagues in the 1970s which renewed interest in the concept of 'non-
sterile immunity' or 'tolerance' to trypanosomes. In other words, a
state in which cattle, after repeated natural challenge, become resistant to the effects of trypanosomiasis although parasites may be
commonly found in their blood. Initially in Uganda Wilson *et al*.
(1975a) studied the performance of a breeding herd introduced and
maintained for 2 years in an area of heavy trypanosome challenge.
Chemotherapy using Berenil was given to animals only on an individual
basis whenever their haematocrit fell below 20% or if they were clinically ill. During the 2 year observation period each animal required
an average of 8 treatments, and became parasitaemic again generally
about 35 days after each treatment. Under this regimen the number of
live calves born increased and subsequent calf mortality decreased;
the incidence of abortion was also reduced.

Even better results were obtained using a similar system of chemotherapy in an area of medium trypanosome challenge in Kenya (Wilson
et al. 1975b, 1976). In this situation steers were introduced and
observed over a 29 month period. Initially the period between drug
treatments was about 50 days, but this increased to around 130 days
by the 9th treatment, and some steers which received no therapy for
the last 6 months of the experiment continued to survive and grow at
a similar rate to those receiving treatment. Control animals which
received no therapy and were introduced at intervals during the
experiment developed signs of severe trypanosomiasis and generally
died. A further group of animals, which were all given Berenil whenever one animal in the group required therapy, continued to require
treatment approximately every 26 days throughout the experiment and
when treatment was withdrawn from some of them for the last 6 month
period, their weight gains were considerably less than those in which
treatment continued.

Studies of the development of non-sterile immunity in endemic areas
have raised several crucial points. First, it is obvious from all
the schemes reported that high levels of veterinary supervision and
cattle husbandry are essential. Secondly, adequate nutrition and
relative freedom from concomitant infections are required (MacLennan
1970; Bourn and Scott 1978). Thirdly, the eradication of tsetse is
not necessarily required before settlement in endemic areas, nor is it
necessary to rely on mechanized farming.

6.5. General conclusions

The examples quoted serve to show that current chemotherapy methods
can be successful in the field, despite the pharmacological problems,

provided adequate funding, staff and facilities are made available. Furthermore, it is interesting that under the schemes described, drug resistance did not emerge as a major problem. In addition, it is apparent that valuable non-sterile immunity can be developed using strategic therapy, though such schemes do require diagnostic facilities and, if these are not available, regular therapy at 2 or 3 monthly intervals is probably more feasible.

Finally, two major inadequacies remain. First, despite the success of many chemotherapy programmes and the millions of doses of drugs uséd each year, there is a serious need for more fully documented field evaluations of different chemotherapy regimens. Secondly, despite the fact that drug resistance can be minimized by careful supervision, adequate dosage and alternate use of available drugs, an additional range of new trypanosomicidal drugs is urgently required to augment the current restricted range of chemotherapeutic agents. Both these problems are beyond the resources of individual countries and therefore require international support from aid agencies and pharmaceutical companies.

6.6. References

Bauer, F. (1958). Über den Wirkungsmechanismus des Berenil (4,4'-Diamidinodiazoamino-benzol) bei *T. congolense*. Zentralblatt für Bakteriologie, Parasitenkunde, Infectionskrankheiten und Hygiene 172, 605-620.

Bevan, Ll.E.W. (1928). A method of inoculating cattle against trypanosomiasis. Transactions of the Royal Society of Tropical Medicine and Hygiene 22, 147-156.

Blaser, E., Jibo, J.M.C. and McIntyre, I. (1979). A field trial of the protective effect of Samorin and Berenil in Zebu cattle under ranching conditions in Tanzania, in Proceedings of the Fifteenth Meeting, International Scientific Council for Trypanosomiasis Research and Control, Banjul, The Gambia, 1977, pp. 384-417. ELEZA Services, Nairobi.

Bourn, D. and Scott, M. (1978). The successful use of work oxen in agricultural development of tsetse infested land in Ethiopia. Tropical Animal Health and Production 10, 191-203.

Braend, M. (1979). World veterinary manpower: comparative aspects. Veterinary Record 105, 77-79.

Davey, D.G. (1957). The chemotherapy of animal trypanosomiasis with particular reference to the trypanosomal diseases of domestic animals in Africa. Veterinary Reviews and Annotations 3, 15-36.

Ford, J. and Blaser, E. (1971). Some aspects of cattle-raising under prophylactic treatment against trypanosomiasis on the Mkwaja Ranch, Tanzania. Acta Tropica 28, 69-79.

Gilbert, R.J. and Newton, B.A. (in press). Studies on the pharmacokinetics of trypanocides with particular reference to Ethidium bromide, in Proceedings of the International Symposium on Nuclear

Techniques in the Study and Control of Parasitic Diseases of Man and Animals, Vienna, 1981. International Atomic Energy Authority, Vienna.

Gilbert, R.J., Curtis, R.J. and Newton, B.A. (1979). The pharmaco-kinetics of (^{14}C)-Ethidium bromide in uninfected and *Trypanosoma congolense* infected calves. Parasitology 79, ii.

Goble, F.C., Fewell, B. and Steiglitz, A.R. (1959). The virulence and drug susceptibility of certain strains of trypanosomes of the Brucei-Evansi group maintained by syringe passage. Annals of Tropical Medicine and Parasitology 53, 189-202.

Goodwin, L.G. and Tierney, E.D. (1977). Trypanocidal activity of blood and tissue fluid from normal and infected rabbits treated with curative drugs. Parasitology 74, 33-45.

Gray, A.R. and Roberts, C.J. (1971). The cyclical transmission of strains of *T. congolense* and *T. vivax* resistant to normal therapeutic doses of trypanocidal drugs. Parasitology 63, 67-89.

Holmes, P.H., Mamo, E., Thomson, A., Knight, P.A., Lucken, R., Murray, P.K., Murray, M., Jennings, F.W. and Urquhart, G.M. (1974). Immunosuppression in bovine trypanosomiasis. Veterinary Record 95, 86-87.

Jahnke, H.E. (1974). The economics of controlling tsetse flies and cattle trypanosomiasis in Africa examined for the case of Uganda. IFO Forschungsberichte der Afrika-Studienstelle 48. Ifo-Institut für Wirtschaftsforschung, Weltforum Verlag, München.

Jennings, F.W., Whitelaw, D.D. and Urquhart, G.M. (1977). The rel-ationship between duration of infection with *Trypanosoma brucei* in mice and the efficacy of chemotherapy. Parasitology 75, 143-153.

Jennings, F.W., Whitelaw, D.D., Holmes, P.H., Chizyuka, H.G.B. and Urquhart, G.M. (1979). The brain as a source of relapsing *Trypanosoma brucei* infection in mice following chemotherapy. International Journal for Parasitology 9, 381-384.

MacLennan, K.J.R. (1970). The epizootiology of trypanosomiasis in livestock in West Africa, in The African Trypanosomiases (edited by H.W. Mulligan), pp. 799-821. George Allen and Unwin, London.

MacLennan, K.J.R. (1971). The aparasitaemic interval following dimin-azine aceturate therapy of a relapsing strain of *T. vivax* infecting cattle. Tropical Animal Health and Production 3, 208-212.

MacLennan, K.J.R. and Na'isa, B.K. (1970). Relapsing *T. vivax* infec-tions in Nigerian Zebu cattle treated with diminazine aceturate. Tropical Animal Health and Production 2, 189-195.

Rüchel, W.-M. (1975). Chemoprophylaxis of bovine trypanosomiasis. Thesis from the Veterinary Institute of the University of Göttingen, published by the German Agency for Technical Co-operation (GTZ), Central Department for Agriculture and Forestry, Eschborn.

Scott, J.M., Pegram, R.G., Holmes, P.H., Pay, T.W.F., Knight, P.A., Jennings, F.W. and Urquhart, G.M. (1977). Immunosuppression in bovine trypanosomiasis: field studies using foot-and-mouth disease vaccine and clostridial vaccine. Tropical Animal Health and Production 9, 159-165.

Stephen, L.E. (1962). Some observations on the behaviour of trypanosomes occurring in cattle previously treated with prophylactic drugs. Annals of Tropical Medicine and Parasitology 56, 415-421.

Van Hoeve, K. and Cunningham, M.P. (1964). Prophylactic activity of Berenil against trypanosomes in treated cattle. Veterinary Record 76, 260.

Whitelaw, D.D., Scott, J.M., Reid, H.W., Holmes, P.H., Jennings, F.W. and Urquhart, G.M. (1979). Immunosuppression in bovine trypanosomiasis: studies with louping-ill vaccine. Research in Veterinary Science 26, 102-107.

Whiteside, E.F. (1962). Interactions between drugs, trypanosomes and cattle in the field, in Drugs, Parasites and Hosts (edited by L.G. Goodwin and R.H. Nimmo-Smith), pp. 116-141. J. and A. Churchill, London.

Williamson, J. (1970). Review of chemotherapeutic and chemoprophylactic agents, in The African Trypanosomiases (edited by H.W. Mulligan), pp. 125-221. George Allen and Unwin, London.

Wilson, A.J., Paris, J. and Dar, F.K. (1975a). Maintenance of a herd of breeding cattle in an area of high trypanosome challenge. Tropical Animal Health and Production 7, 63-71.

Wilson, A.J., Le Roux, T.G., Paris, J., Davidson, C.R. and Gray, A.R. (1975b). Observations on a herd of beef cattle maintained in a tsetse area. I. Assessment of chemotherapy as a method of the control of trypanosomiasis. Tropical Animal Health and Production 7, 187-199.

Wilson, A.J., Paris, J., Luckins, A.G., Dar, F.K. and Gray, A.R. (1976). Observations on a herd of beef cattle maintained in a tsetse area. II. Assessment of the development of immunity in association with trypanocidal drug treatment. Tropical Animal Health and Production 8, 1-12.

CHAPTER 7
The Problem of Chagas's Disease Vector Control

C.J. Schofield

Department of Entomology,
London School of Hygiene and Tropical Medicine,
Keppel Street,
London, WC1E 7HT.

7.1. Introduction

   With a few exceptions, most countries in Latin America have invested
time and resources into research and control campaigns aimed at reducing
or eliminating domestic populations of triatomine bugs and thus reducing
the risk of Chagas's disease transmission. This effort, supported by
many international organizations such as WHO, PAHO and the Wellcome
Trust, has produced several hundred scientific publications but only
a few qualified success stories - in Bambuí, Minas Gerais, and parts
of São Paulo State, Brazil, and also parts of Argentina. Several
other campaigns, smaller in size and duration, have also met with a
degree of success in other parts of Latin America. In spite of this,
a high incidence of domestic vectors remains in most of the tradition-
ally endemic areas, and some domestic vectors such as *Triatoma infestans*
seem to be expanding their geographic distribution (Barrett *et al*.
1979; Ormerod 1979).

   Any campaign of Chagas's disease control should include interruption
of transmission, specifically by eliminating the vectors, yet the
amount of research into vectors and their control now seems dispro-
ortionately small compared to research along less immediately fruitful
lines such as immunology. Analysis of research projects on Chagas's
disease funded by the State Secretariat for Science and Technology
(SECYT) of Argentina in 1979-1980 showed that 46% were on parasite
immunology and biochemistry, 25% on clinical studies (including chemotherapy), 9% on congenital Chagas's disease, and 20% on vector research.
Perhaps part of the reason for this arises from the idea that although
vectors should be controlled, they are not, and so an alternative must
be provided. As Brener (1980) points out, much of the interest in
vaccination stems from a certain disenchantment with vector control.

   Some would point out that existing methods of vector control are
powerful enough, but they are simply not being applied correctly,

adequately, widely, or frequently enough. Exponents of this view emphasise administrative, organizational and financial problems, but it would be unfair to confine criticism to any inertia of the health services and it is fruitless to do so without trying to see what can be done to help.

7.2. The problems

7.2.1. Planning

Prescott (1979) has emphasised that we have as yet no economic just-ification for any particular level of investment in control. In assigning priorities for research, this is a handicap, and some sort of economic analysis should therefore be undertaken in order to justify requisite levels of funding and to provide a framework for selecting the most cost-effective approach to vector control.

7.2.2. Logistics

The logistic problems are a little more tangible. The area under consideration is vast, but except for coastal areas, is typified by dry savanna-like plains with a low level of agricultural development and a widely dispersed rural population, often with difficult access to main routes of communication (Figure 1). Often, the rural pop-ulations are poorly documented and existing maps may be quite inaccurate. Whatever system of control is to be applied, the same logistic prob-lems must be faced, and there is an obvious need for some sort of net-work analysis to help optimize control delivery.

One approach, practised widely in Brazil, involves a huge effort to map and survey the affected areas, pinpointing infested houses, and planning a wide-reaching campaign eventually to spray each house with insecticides, followed by selective spraying of re-emergent infest-ations (SUCAM 1980). Given the special circumstances of the Brazilian interior, and the current development policy which includes the con-struction of many new roads, this plan is clearly advantageous, although the large expenditure on transport poses considerable difficulties.

An alternative approach, being examined in Argentina, considers the possibility of first concentrating the widely dispersed populations in new rural townships. The vast Argentine chaco, which has the highest incidence of Chagas's disease in the country, is a dry region which has suffered intense over-exploitation during the last 50 years. The process of land degradation, through overgrazing and excessive timbering, is fairly well understood (Figure 2). It has resulted in immense areas of unproductive thornscrub, interrupted by stretches of barren land around extremely poor settlements (ranchos) dedicated mainly to rearing goats. In one part of the province of Salta however, this process has been reversed by careful land management which in-cluded concentrating the widely-dispersed human population in a new township based on an emerging timber, charcoal, and cattle industry. As a result, basic services to the community such as primary education

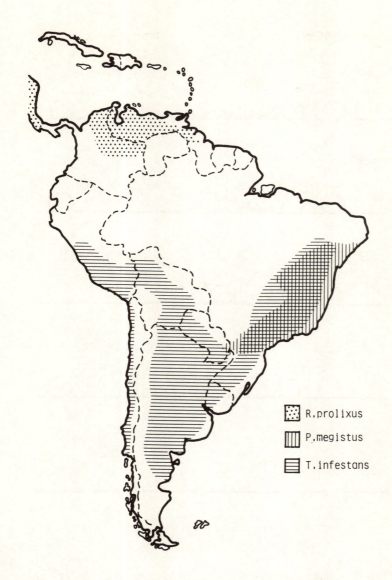

Figure 1. Approximate distribution of the three main vectors of Chagas's disease in South America: *Rhodnius prolixus*, *Panstrongylus megistus* and *Triatoma infestans*. Not shown are *Triatoma dimidiata*, important in Central America, Columbia and Ecuador, and *Triatoma braziliensis*, important in the dry northeast of Brazil.

74

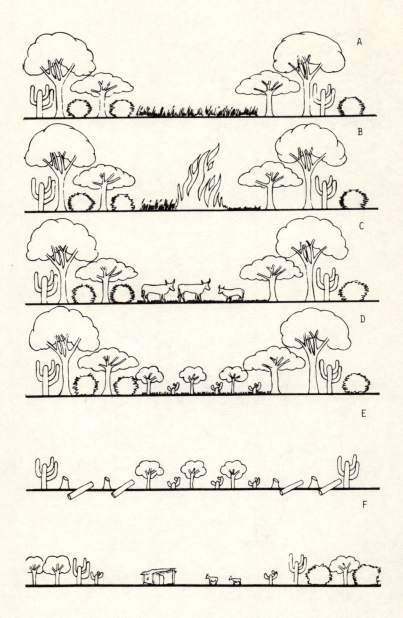

Figure 2.   The process of land degradation in the Argentine chaco.
(Continued on next page.)

and health-care can be provided and, whenever necessary, vector control by house-spraying can be carried out in a few days rather than the several months required if the population had remained dispersed. In this way many of the logistic difficulties of control have been over-come, and it is to be hoped that this sensible approach to land-management linked to disease control will prove applicable to other areas (Bucher and Schofield 1981).

7.2.3. Control methods

For some, pragmatists, the choice of control method is dictated by which products are available on international or national markets. For others, the choice is more emotive and includes rural development, public health education, and housing improvements. Bearing in mind the existing structure and expertise of vector control organizations, it seems likely that the most effective plan will include elements of both viewpoints. Table 1 summarizes existing and potential control options.

Existing control methods, particularly high dosage spraying of BHC, do work under certain circumstances, but this approach is somewhat empirical. After spraying, we can expect a bug population to fall, probably to below detectable levels. But what happens then? Does that population go extinct or does it survive at low levels? If small residual populations remain do they constitute a real threat for disease transmission?

The problem for vector control is that, at some time after spraying, bug populations are likely to re-emerge to detectable levels and, if

---

Figure 2. (Continued.) The chaco is a huge outwash plain built up mainly of sediments from the eastern Andes. The climate is arid and primary minerals and soluble salts are abundant. The heavy textured soils make the area susceptible to flooding during the wet season, and low areas with poor drainage have extensive salt pans. The original vegetation of the chaco is a mosaic of woodland and grass-land (A). Grassland is protected from encroaching woodland by periodic fires (B), which maintain a stable mosaic. Although this ecosystem can support a reasonable number of cattle, overgrazing leads to an absence of grass dry matter and to soil erosion (C). Reduction of fires due to the absence of dry grass fuel triggers rapid encroachment by woody vegetation (D). Timbering eliminates large trees, leaving unproductive shrubs and old diseased trees (E). Reduced grassland makes the area unsuitable for cattle and many farmers turn to goats. The goats destroy young trees as well as grasses leaving an impoverished landscape dominated by dense unprod-uctive shrubland where only scattered huts surrounded by barren land remain (F). The poor quality huts and their associated goat corrals are an ideal habitat for *Triatoma infestans*, and the dispersion of the huts exacerbates the logistic problems of Chagas's disease con-trol. (From Bucher and Schofield 1981; reproduced by kind permission of New Scientist.)

Table 1. Chagas's disease vector control.

Insecticides *e.g.*   BHC, Malathion, Fenitrothion, Propoxur, Permethrin.

  Advantages: Cheap, effective, readily available.
  Disadvantages: Loss of residual activity on alkaline porous mud walls.

Insect Growth Regulators *e.g.*   Juvenile hormone mimics, precocenes.

  Advantages: Fairly specific*, safe to mammals.
  Disadvantages: Slow acting, active only on few stages.

Insect Pathogens *e.g.*   *Neoaplectana, Metarrhizium.*

  Advantages: Safe to mammals.
  Disadvantages: Climatic limitations, untested in field, probably expensive.

Biological Control *e.g. Telenomus fariai, Ooencyrtus trinidadensis.*

  Advantages: Safe to mammals.
  Disadvantages: Ineffective in field trials; expensive.

Genetic Control *e.g.*   Release of sterile or sub-sterile males.

  Advantages: None.
  Disadvantages: Unacceptable to release potential vectors; expensive.

Traps *e.g.*   Baited with light, pheromones, kairomones.

  Advantages: None.
  Disadvantages: Ineffective.

Housing Modifications *e.g.*   Wall-plaster, tile or tin roofs.

  Advantages: Effective, general improvement in living standards.
  Disadvantages: Tend to be expensive; climatic problems.

Health Education *e.g.*   Increased public awareness/acceptance; vigilance schemes.

  Advantages: Effective, general improvement in living standards.
  Disadvantages: Increased expectations may not always be fulfilled.

---

* The specificity of insect growth regulators may be disadvantageous since it results in only a small market for commercial products, which may not therefore be economically feasible.

untreated, eventually recover to former levels unless some permanent modification of the domestic habitat has been made. But where do these re-emergent populations come from? Are they from post-spray survivors or are they immigrants from some focus which escaped treatment?

It is important to answer this question because if the problem is mainly from survivors then the answer will involve improvement of spray application, more residual compounds and more frequent respraying. But if the problem arises from immigrants then a more thorough geographic coverage is indicated. With *T. infestans* this may simply require a more thorough treatment of houses, but with vectors with residual sylvatic habitats, such as *R. prolixus*, control of sylvatic foci such as palm trees may be indicated.

Reliance on insecticides, particularly organochlorines, stems partly from tradition (BHC has been in use for some 30 years) and the fact that the infrastructure and expertise for their application already exists. There is thus a certain inertia, an inbuilt resistance to change, particularly since more modern insecticides tend to be considerably more expensive, and the organization required for other methods has not yet been developed on a large scale. However, BHC is becoming relatively scarce, as more countries restrict its use due to concern about environmental pollution and its unpleasant toxicological properties, and its price is increasing. In Latin American countries which have restricted BHC, such as Argentina, carbamates and organophosphates have been used, although their relatively short persistence on mud walls makes them less than ideal substitutes. Synthetic pyrethroids, such as permethrin, have shown good residual effects in field trials and, although they tend to be more than 10 times the price of BHC, less frequent application may make them more cost-effective in the longer term.

Control based on insect growth regulators or pathogens has yet to be effectively demonstrated in the field. However one should not rule out their possible inclusion with other methods. For example, insecticides tend to be least effective against fifth-stage nymphs, whereas juvenile hormone mimics are only really effective against fifth-stages; joint application of the two might therefore be appropriate (Pinchin *et al.* 1978). It is unlikely that biological or genetic control or traps will be of use in controlling triatomine bugs. However, both health education and housing improvements have been shown to be extremely effective and should in any case be pursued as part of general development objectives (Dias and Garcia 1978; Dias and Dias in press; Gamboa 1973; Schofield and Marsden in press).

7.3. Vector response

The choice of control methods, or overall control strategy, depends very much on predicting the response of target vector populations within the temporal and spatial scale of the control. In principle, vector control assumes that bug populations are at a particular level, and attempts to reduce them to either (1) a sustainable lower level,

or (2) extinction. Assuming both alternatives to be practical the
choice of strategy is then dependent on cost and on effectiveness in
reducing transmission of Chagas's disease. I emphasize again that our
understanding of both aspects is inadequate.

How do bug populations respond to changes in density? Although this
is not entirely clear, there are some pointers (Figure 3). Field
data available for *T. infestans* seem to indicate an element of annual
stability in established domestic bug populations, regulated by the
availability of blood sources (Schofield 1980a,b; Schofield and Marsden
1980; and unpublished data). The density of the population is set by
the number of eggs, nymphs, and adults. As density increases in a
stable domestic environment, the nutritional status of adults and
nymphs declines due to mutual interference and competition for blood
meals. Reduced nutritional status leads to increased stage development
times and reduced egg laying, both of which reduce the rate of recruit-
ment to successive stages thus slowing the rate of growth of the population and restoring bug density (relative to available hosts) to its
stable level. Reduced nutritional status can also affect population
density directly by triggering flight by adults. Conversely, a reduction in density can result in improved nutritional status for the
survivors, triggering accelerated population growth leading to recovery
of the population. This mechanism of density regulation functions
within upper and lower limits set by climatic factors, particularly
temperature.

If space becomes severely limited, for example by plastering over
all the cracks and other bug refuges in a house, then bug density may
be reduced through increased exposure to predators such as chickens
and lizards. Normally, however, nutritional requirements limit the
bug populations before this type of predation becomes important.

A simple model of the relationship between density and nutritional
status derives from the more primitive state (*e.g.* of a silvatic bug)
in which the hosts (*e.g.* small rodents) are also predators of the bugs.
Predation (P) is proportional to the number of bugs (D) and their
contact time with the host, *i.e.* the number of feeds taken (f) and the
time spent feeding (t):

$$P = fn \ (D \times f \times t)$$

In order to minimize predation, any increase in density must be acc-
ompanied by a decrease in number of feeds and/or time spent feeding,
both of which lead to reduced nutritional status.

From this understanding, some things are immediately apparent. For
example, education has a vital role to play if affected people can be
encouraged to keep domestic animals outside the house and thus reduce
the availability of food for the bugs. More importantly, it can be
seen that any reduction in bug density due to a short-lived insecticide will tend to promote more rapid reproduction of the survivors
leading to recovery of the population (Figure 4). As bug populations
recover, adult dispersal becomes more important leading to a 'snowball'

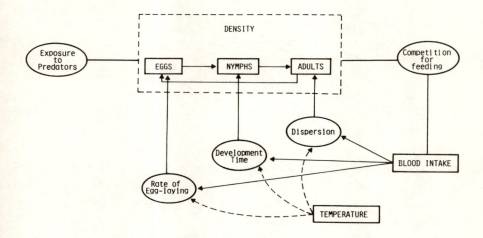

Figure 3. Schematic representation of density regulation in populations of *Triatoma infestans* (see text).

effect increasing the rate of re-emergence of domestic infestations.

Can we predict this and thus plan control campaigns which take into account bug population behaviour, and can we then develop rational comparisons of the cost-effectiveness of different approaches over various time scales?

7.4. Interacting factors

Figure 5 is a crude summary of interacting factors linked particularly to insecticide control. Much neglected is an analysis of costs linked to some appropriate measure of effectiveness (such as 'house-years of infestation prevented', proposed by N.M. Prescott). Equally neglected are the 'externalities' of control, external costs and benefits such as the generation of local employment or partial control of other vectors, which might discount some of the costs of each control strategy and could be of crucial importance in decision-making. I would also highlight the following specific subjects requiring better understanding.

7.4.1. Insecticide characteristics

Triatomine bugs generally have a high tolerance to organic insecticides, and bugs may reproduce for several days in a treated house before succumbing to a lethal dose. The cryptic habits of the bugs

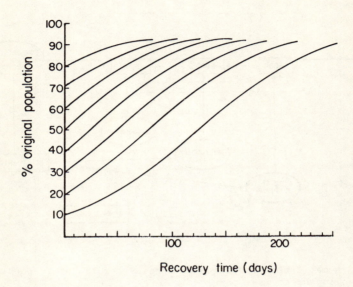

Figure 4. Hypothetical recovery times of *Triatoma infestans* pop-
lation after an instantaneous kill. The curves are derived from a
simple logistic equation $\left[dN/dt = rN(1{-}N/K)\right]$ with the instantaneous
rate of growth of the population (r) set at 0.018. Thus:

$$t = \frac{\ln\left(\frac{K}{N_o} - 1\right) - \ln\left(\frac{K}{N_t} - 1\right)}{r}$$

Where K = carrying capacity (in this case, 100%)
N_t = percentage of original population at time t days
N_o = percentage of original population at time 0 (*i.e.*
% survivors after treatment)

and the protection afforded particularly by densely thatched roofs
mean that even high-dosage spraying with motorized mist-blowers may
fail to reach all the bugs' hiding places. Some insecticides have
repellent effects which may cause bugs to remain hidden in their refuges for several weeks, during which time the activity of the insecticide may decline sharply. We have insufficient knowledge of the
degree of coverage and penetration of house walls and roofs during a
typical spray routine, and we need to know more about the rate of fall-
off in activity of the insecticides on porous mud walls under the
extreme climatic conditions found in many parts of Latin America. With

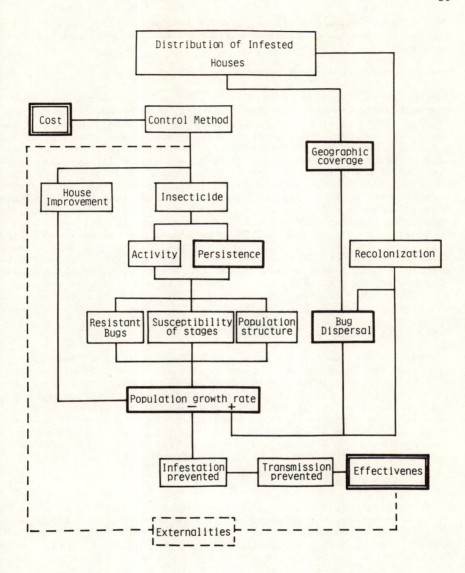

Figure 5.   Summary of interacting factors concerned with insecticide
treatment of triatomine bugs. Heavily outlined boxes emphasize
areas requiring better understanding.

this information we may arrive at reasonable predictions about the time course of exposure to lethal insecticides experienced by the bug population.

7.4.2. Population growth rates

Although well studied in the laboratory, the behaviour of bug populations under natural conditions is poorly understood. Only the crudest estimates of natural mortality have been made, and most of its causes are unknown. To make reasonable predictions of bug population behaviour in response to treatment it is important to predict at least nett changes in bug numbers according to population density and structure, and also to understand the role of seasonal and daily fluctuations in temperature and humidity in regulating these changes. Unfortunately, even the natural microclimate to which bugs are exposed inside infested houses is poorly documented. The excellent work of Kroeger (1980), monitoring temperature fluctuations in modern and traditional houses in Ecuador, should be repeated in other areas, particularly the cooler regions of Argentina and Chile. The typical 'rancho' of these areas seems to smooth out daily temperature fluctuations, but minimum temperatures can drop well below 15°C on cold nights even though charcoal braziers may be lit inside the houses. It is not known to what extent these low night-time temperatures reduce bug reproduction during the winter months.

7.4.3. Bug dispersal

Bugs can be dispersed actively through adult flight (Lehane and Schofield 1981) and passively through carriage by man and other vertebrates (Schofield 1979). We do not know the relative importance of these mechanisms, nor the degree to which they contribute to bug population growth either in individual houses or over a geographic area. From laboratory observations we can predict the proportion of adults likely to fly from a population of known nutritional status (Lehane and Schofield, unpublished), but it is unclear how far they will go, and a complete mystery as to which direction they will take.

7.4.4. Geographic coverage

If bug dispersal is, as we suspect, a major source of recolonization of treated houses, it becomes vital to know more about the geographic distribution of houses, the rate at which they can be treated, and the likely proportion of houses which will escape treatment. This latter figure, assumed to be zero by optimists, has been put as high as 20% by pessimists in difficult areas. Some study of this question is obviously indicated, both to identify reasons for poor coverage and also to assess the likely importance of untreated houses as sources for recolonizing bugs. For example, if houses are missed because they are extremely isolated, they may pose little threat to recolonize treated houses; but if they are missed because of poor public acceptance of the treatment, steps must be taken to improve this.

7.5. Conclusions

An outstanding problem is the fragmentary nature of research, knowledge and opinion. There is an obvious need for an interdisciplinary
approach using modern methods of systems analysis, to compare different approaches to control over specified geographic areas within
stated constraints of acceptable levels of control and acceptable
levels of expenditure. This should include full cooperation with
governments so that realistic decision-making criteria can be defined
within existing government policies. I have tried to highlight what
seem to be obvious uncertainties in our knowledge, but the relative
importance of these aspects is really based on my own experience and
opinions rather than on a truly systematic analysis of the vector
control problem. Although existing control techniques can be used
to control the problem, the available tools need to be united in a
clear overall plan. A recent attempt to integrate the wide range of
experience of Chagas's disease control in Venezuela, using an adaptive
management approach, was perhaps a first step towards the necessary
interdisciplinary view of Chagas's disease in general. This workshop
combined entomologists, epidemiologists, control specialists, sociol-
ogists, immunologists and biochemists. The resulting simulation of
various control strategies showed that even with optimistic assumptions
about their efficiency, neither chemotherapy nor vaccination provided
satisfactory decline in transmission risk over a 20 year period. Only
vector control through insecticides and/or house improvement predicted
a satisfactory decline in disease transmission (Rabinovich 1981,
unpublished report to WHO). Perhaps some realignment of research and
control priorities is indicated?

Acknowledgements

I thank my colleagues Enrique Bucher of the Centro de Zoologia
Aplicada, Córdoba, and Richard Pinchin formerly of the Universidade
Federal de Rio de Janeiro, for their help and encouragement.
Financial support from the Wellcome Trust is gratefully acknowledged.

7.6. References

Barrett, T.V., Hoff, R., Mott, K.E., Guedes, F. and Sherlock, I.A.
   (1979). An outbreak of acute Chagas's disease in the São Francisco
   valley region of Bahia, Brazil: triatomine vectors and animal
   reservoirs of *Trypanosoma cruzi*. Transactions of the Royal Society
   of Tropical Medicine and Hygiene 73, 703-709.

Brener, Z. (1980). Vacinação, in *Trypanosoma cruzi* e doença de Chagas
   (edited by Z. Brener and Z.A. Andrade), pp. 450-455. Editora
   Guanabara Koogan, Rio de Janeiro.

Bucher, E.H. and Schofield, C.J. (1981). Economic assault on Chagas
   disease. New Scientist, 29 October 1981, 321-324.

Dias, J.C.P. and Garcia, A.L.R. (1978). Vigilância epidemiológica con participación comunitária. Un programa de enfermedad de Chagas. Boletin de la Oficina Sanitaria Panamericana 84, 533-544.

Dias, J.C.P. and Dias, R.B. (in press). Participação da comunidade em programas de controle da doença de Chagas. Boletin de la Oficina Sanitaria Panamericana.

Gamboa, C.J. (1973). El processo modificador de la vivienda en el medio rural del estado Miranda (Venezuela). Su relación con la infestación por *Rhodnius prolixus*. Archivos Venezolanos de Medicina Tropical y Parasitologia Medica 5, 353-364.

Kroeger, A. (1980). Housing and health in the process of cultural adaptation: a case study among jungle and highland natives of Ecuador. Journal of Tropical Medicine and Hygiene 83, 53-69.

Lehane, M.J. and Schofield, C.J. (1981). Field experiments of dispersive flight by *Triatoma infestans*. Transactions of the Royal Society of Tropical Medicine and Hygiene 75, 399-400.

Ormerod, W.E. (1979). Human and animal trypanosomiases as world health problems. Pharmacology and Therapeutics 6, 1-40.

Pinchin, R., Oliveira Filho, A.M.de, Figueiredo, M.J., Muller, C.A. and Gilbert, B. (1978). Slow release juvenile hormone formulations for triatomine control. Transactions of the Royal Society of Tropical Medicine and Hygiene 72, 322-323.

Prescott, N.M. (1979). The economics of malaria, filariases and human trypanosomiasis. World Health Organization unpublished report, TDR/SER/SC-1/80.4.

Schofield, C.J. (1979). The behaviour of Triatominae (Hemiptera: Reduviidae): a review. Bulletin of Entomological Research 69, 363-379.

Schofield, C.J. (1980a). Density regulation of domestic populations of *Triatoma infestans* in Brazil. Transactions of the Royal Society of Tropical Medicine and Hygiene 74, 761-769.

Schofield, C.J. (1980b). Nutritional status of domestic populations of *Triatoma infestans*. Transactions of the Royal Society of Tropical Medicine and Hygiene 74, 770-778.

Schofield, C.J. and Marsden, P.D. (in press). The effect of wall plaster on a domestic population of *Triatoma infestans*. Bulletin of the Pan American Health Organization (also reproduced as World Health Organization mimeographed report no. WHO/VBC/80.757.)

SUCAM (1980). Manual de Normas Technicas de Campanha de Controle da Doença de Chagas. Superintendencia da Campanha Anti-Malaria, Ministerio da Saúde, Brasilia.

CHAPTER 8
Trends in Research on Tsetse Biology

D.H. Molyneux

Department of Biology,
University of Salford,
Salford, M5 4WT.

8.1. Introduction

This paper assesses our current knowledge of the biology of *Glossina*
in relation to control and appraises the areas where advances relevant
to control could be made. The material presented will be necessarily
selective. Before defining inadequacies it is necessary to highlight
areas where advances have been made which show promise for the future,
for only by pursuing these can progress towards solutions of the field
problems be achieved.

Glossina species have been the targets of a variety of control
operations since they were identified as the vectors of human and
animal trypanosomiases early in this century (see reviews on *Glossina*
as vectors by Jordan 1974, 1976; Molyneux 1977). Initial efforts at
control depended on the modification of habitat by bush clearing or
removing the host game animals. Bush clearing was either total or
partial, the latter especially in areas where riverine flies were
transmitting the human disease and where riverine vegetation clearance
destroyed the habitat of *G. palpalis* and *G. tachinoides*. In epidemics
of sleeping sickness in East Africa, population movement away from
fly-infested areas was adopted to reduce man-fly contact, and thus
transmission (Ford 1971). It is important to emphasize the different
objectives which tsetse control has in relation to human and animal
trypanosomiasis. In human trypanosomiasis vector control measures
are instituted to reduce epidemic transmission of disease and allow
medical services time to identify and treat cases through surveillance
teams; vector control is unlikely to be cost effective in endemic
sleeping sickness. In animal trypanosomiasis control or eradication
has a different, economic objective: to allow livestock to become
productive in areas where previously they were not. Eradication (in
a defined local situation) is frequently an economically justifiable
but long-term pursuit, whereas control may not be. Change of goal
from eradication to control reduces or abolishes the potential economic

benefits. Programmes may be justifiable, however, if they are to
prevent extension of fly belts, particularly of *G. morsitans* (MacLennan
1981). It is increasingly recognized that tsetse control should be
combined with planned land use (Jordan 1978, 1979; MacLennan 1981;
FAO 1981). It is against this background that tsetse biology and
control research should be assessed.

A major impetus to *Glossina* control came from the introduction of
insecticides, initially DDT. The spectacular results obtained in
South Africa (du Toit 1954) and subsequently maintained in Nigeria
over a long period (Davies 1964, 1971) testify to the effectiveness of
simple techniques on a large scale provided adequate logistic support
is available. The techniques of ground spray application developed
over several years depended on the persistence of the insecticide and
its economic use by selective and discriminative application. As
costs (of both labour and chemicals) rose, techniques became more refined and, with the development of aerial application, less labour
intensive. Meanwhile, environmentalists were concerned at the contamination of the natural ecosystem by chlorinated hydrocarbons, following the demonstration of side effects of these pesticides; although,
in terms of kilograms of pesticide per unit area, tsetse control contributes relatively little to the total amount of insecticide applied.
Even in Africa, where indiscriminate agricultural use of pesticides is
rarely monitored, concern was expressed that tsetse control by insecticide could damage ecosystems, and detailed studies of its effects on
non-target organisms were proposed. The development of sequential
non-residual application of insecticides using fixed wing aircraft has
reduced contamination and allowed large areas to be treated.

Increasing sophistication of modern aerial spraying technology and
increasing fuel and insecticide costs have provoked a search for more
cost effective techniques which can be operated by the community,
initiating a trend towards simpler, passive methods of control. At
the same time, studies on the ecology, behaviour and physiology of
Glossina have opened the way to new potential techniques based on
trapping using olfactory attractants.

Environmental concern, the success of sterile insect release (SIR)
in control of screwworm (*Cochliomyia hominivorax*) in the United States,
and the problems of insecticide application in more humid zones, all
stimulated research into mass rearing of *Glossina* with the objective
of testing SIR. After several years' investigation it appears that
the technique can eradicate *G. palpalis gambiensis* in a limited linear
habitat, though more extensive trials are required.

Much progress has been made in various areas of tsetse biology.
Optimistically, it could be stated (1) there is as yet no recorded
resistance to insecticides; (2) the synthetic pyrethroids could replace the chlorinated hydrocarbons, if necessary; (3) environmental
sequelae of the pesticides in use are known, and (4) more promising
developments using low cost techniques or techniques based on olfactory
attraction and autosterilization are in prospect. Inadequacies

appear however not at the scientific, but at the operational level.
The need is to identify the problem, and then to create the organization and seek the finance needed to solve it with currently available
tools, whilst undertaking research and exploiting new findings relevant to control. An attempt is made to review recent work in this
paper. Work reviewed earlier (*e.g.* by Mulligan 1970; Jordan 1974,
1978; FAO 1977; Laird 1977) will not be cited unless relevant to more
recent studies.

8.2. Insecticides, their application and side-effects

8.2.1. Non-residual application by helicopter

The introduction of synthetic pyrethroids (Elliott *et al.* 1978) was
followed by small scale field trials of these pesticides for the control of *Glossina*. Non-residual sequential application as aerosols of
these compounds, particularly permethrin and deltamethrin (formerly
decamethrin), showed considerable promise (Molyneux *et al.* 1978; Van
Wettere *et al.* 1978; Baldry *et al.* 1978). The pyrethroids were applied by helicopter to riverine forest in the northern Guinea savanna
vegetation zone of West Africa, against *G. tachinoides* and *G. palpalis*
sspp. Molyneux *et al.* (1978) summarized the results obtained with
six insecticides at dosages equivalent to 5 and 10g active ingredient
(a.i.) of endosulfan per hectare, calculated from topical application
studies in the laboratory. The details of equipment used and its
calibration, as well as meteorological studies, were described by Lee
et al. (1978). During these trials a unilateral application technique,
with rotary atomizers placed on one side of the helicopter, was developed and subsequently used (Baldry *et al.* 1978, 1981).

Aerosol application with dosage as low as $0.19g(a.i.)ha^{-1}$ and $0.36g$
$(a.i.)ha^{-1}$ of deltamethrin reduced *G. tachinoides* populations by up
to 98.5% of non-teneral male flies and 78.5% of females; permethrin in
sequential applications did not perform as well as deltamethrin;
endosulfan at 5.4g and $9.0g(a.i.)ha^{-1}$ reduced populations by between
90-98%. All populations were monitored by white biconical traps
(Challier and Laveissière 1973).

The results achieved by deltamethrin at such low dosages were confirmed by Van der Vloedt *et al.* (1980) and could have been due to the
'knockdown' effect recently described by Quinlan and Gatehouse (1981a).
The likelihood of a 'knocked-down' *Glossina* surviving predation is
very small.

The most promising organophosphate (fenthion) did not perform in
field trials as well as had been hoped. However, unlike other pesticides in use against *Glossina*, fenthion is more effective against old
pregnant females than younger flies (both male and female tenerals).
Thus it may have advantages in integrated control, as the pregnant
females are those least susceptible to endosulfan and the pyrethroids.
Incorporation of fenthion into some kind of combined sequential application could be an appropriate strategy.

8.2.2. Residual application by helicopter

Residual applications of endosulfan, dieldrin and DDT either by ground spray methods (see FAO 1977) or, more recently, by helicopter have been important methods of control over the past 30 years. In Nigeria, helicopter (Bell 47G) applications, using initially boom and nozzle equipment, at dosages of 1500g ha^{-1} of endosulfan and 500g ha^{-1} of dieldrin, controlled *G. m. submorsitans* for several months. Later trials using rotary atomizers suggested *Glossina* was exterminated by dosages of 640g ha^{-1} dieldrin and 800g ha^{-1} endosulfan to 10% of the area infested by fly (FAO 1977). Speilberger *et al*. (1979) obtained most promising results by the application of synthetic pyrethroids (deltamethrin, permethrin and cypermethrin) in sprays, using droplets of 150 μm volume mean diameter (VMD) to give a residual deposit; they eradicated the riverine species with a single application of deltamethrin at a dosage of 30g(a.i.) ha^{-1} and suggested that similar results could be achieved using a 200g ha^{-1} permethrin wettable powder formulation and by cypermethrin at 150g ha^{-1}.

Lee *et al*. (1980) and Baldry *et al*. (1981) attempted to reduce dosages of endosulfan and permethrin. Good results were achieved with 100g and 200g ha^{-1} of endosulfan and 50g ha^{-1} permethrin wettable powder.

8.2.3. Fixed wing aerosol application techniques

Use of the fixed wing aerosol technique has been extensively studied for control or eradication of *G. m. centralis* in Botswana and Zambia, and *G. m. morsitans* in Zambia and Zimbabwe. Endosulfan has been most frequently used at dosages of 10-15g ha^{-1}; recently deltamethrin has been tried on a small scale. This technique requires a flat terrain. The method now employs twin engined aircraft (*e.g.* Beechcraft Baron or Piper Aztec), and is usually carried out at night using navigation aids and flying at 280 km hr^{-1} in parallel paths 200-300 m apart, producing swathes of 100-300 metres. Droplet sizes of 30-35 μm VMD are optimal, using endosulfan at 6-12g ha^{-1}. Inversion conditions are essential for all types of aerial application; although night flying provides the most suitable meteorological condition, it is not feasible using a helicopter or over difficult terrain. Thus in many situations it is possible to spray only early in the morning and just before nightfall. It is essential to monitor meteorological conditions to assess the most suitable times for application in areas where night flying is not possible (Lee 1977). In the more humid conditions of forest and preforest zones inversion conditions may not exist at all, and hence aerial spray application may not be feasible.

Sequential applications of non-residual insecticides should be acc-ompanied by detailed evaluation of the density and age structure of the tested populations. Ovarian ageing (Challier 1965) of flies remaining after spraying can determine the efficacy of the application and provide information on reinvasion or insecticide drift (Davies 1981). Ovarian ageing is also necessary to determine the time between

successful applications (related to inter-larval period) and the
number of spray cycles to be applied, so that the last spray will kill
adults emerging from pupae deposited immediately before the first
cycle began (Davies 1978).

There is little available detailed information on two fixed wing
applications carried out in Nigeria and Ivory Coast. The terrain in
each area was not suitable for night flying and details of entomological evaluation are not yet available. Further detailed and controlled
studies on the fixed wing technique in West Africa savanna habitats
are required.

8.2.4. Possibility of insecticide resistance

There is no recorded insecticide resistance in *Glossina* yet. However,
Maudlin *et al.* (1981) developed a computer model which predicted the
development of resistance if repeated application of the same insecticide was made at long intervals. These workers also identified DDE,
a breakdown product of DDT, in *Glossina* treated with DDT. This suggests,
if the system is similar to that in other insects, that DDT-susceptible
tsetse must have the gene for producing DDT-ase. Thus, although
insecticide resistance has yet to develop in *Glossina*, it could occur.
The effects of sublethal doses of endosulfan in the laboratory have
been studied by Quinlan and Gatehouse (1981b), and Davies (1981) described the effect of insecticide drift on *G. m. centralis* populations
in Botswana. Aerosol application of 6-12g ha^{-1} endosulfan had an
effect 20 km downwind. The reduction of the population varied with
the distance from the sprayed area. However, as some old females survived 5 or 6 applications, it is possible that downwind drift could
result in the development of insecticide resistance.

Although it is not strictly related to insecticide resistance,
Golder and Patel (1980) suggested that *Glossina* infected with *T. brucei*
and showing changes in salivary gland structure and biochemistry are
more susceptible to endosulfan applied topically than uninfected flies,
possibly due to the effects of the trypanosomes on acetylcholinesterase
distribution. This suggestion merits further study.

8.2.5. Environmental monitoring of effects of insecticide

Considerable concern has been expressed about the side effects of
pesticide application. Attempts have been made to develop less environmentally contaminative application methods, to be selective in
choosing the pesticide and economical in its application. Koeman *et
al.* (1980) reviewed the environmental consequences of using insecticides in *Glossina* control and established criteria governing their
use. It is now clear which insecticides should be chosen in particular
habitats, what the expected mortality will be in particular faunal
groups and which indicator species or families are most susceptible to
particular insecticides. The numbers of an animal species should not
be reduced by the pesticide dose to a level at which their survival in
a particular area would be endangered, and disequilibria or severe

shifts in relative abundance should not occur. Compounds accumulating in the food web should be avoided. Although acute effects undoubtedly occur, the change of land use associated with development, including wholesale habitat destruction, following effective tsetse control causes much more serious and long term effects than a single pesticide application. Attempts to minimize environmental impact in large scale operations should therefore be made, including (1) assessment of the effects spraying has on the fauna, particularly in relation to local traditions, sources of protein and the likely loss of potential wildlife refuges; (2) attempts to apply insecticides as discriminatively as possible *e.g.* by combining ground or aerial spraying with sterile male release; (3) if possible, use of least contaminative methods such as sequential aerosols which cause little damage to vertebrates; and (4) leaving unsprayed areas from which natural fauna could reoccupy sprayed habitats.

Even sequential low doses of endosulfan (6-12g(a.i.)ha^{-1} per application), applied in the Okavango delta of Botswana, produced sublethal and reversible effects on the fish populations. Erythrocyte and leucocyte counts, haemoglobin and plasma protein levels changed during spraying but returned to normal, pre-spray, values within six months and pathological changes occurred in the liver and brain of fish at the onset of spraying; also, in sprayed areas the 'nesting' behaviour of *Tilapia rendalli* was disturbed and 'nest' building reduced by 75% compared with unsprayed areas (Mattheissen 1981). However, no effect of 3 years spraying could be detected by detailed longitudinal studies of freshwater invertebrate populations (Russell-Smith and Ruckert 1981). There has been considerable increase over the last decade in knowledge of the effects of pesticide on non-target organisms. Despite justifiable expressions of concern about the environmental effects of these compounds, the quantities used and the extent of *Glossina* control in Africa are very small compared with the quantities of chlorinated hydrocarbon used in cotton spraying, where up to 70 kg ha^{-1} may be applied annually; little outcry accompanies this continual application of pesticide at levels 50 times greater than those used in *Glossina* control (Chapin and Wasserstrom 1981). There seems little need therefore at present for further studies on environmental effects; suitable dosages and methods of application in particular habitats are defined, and the likely consequences known. There is also seemingly little that can be done to protect tropical Africa from the degradation of the fuelwood industry (Roche 1975; Moss and Morgan 1981), the environmental consequences of which have yet to be fully assessed in relation to tsetse and trypanosomiasis.

8.3. Novel and potential control methods

8.3.1. Insect growth regulators

Insect growth regulators (IGRs) interfere with chitin synthesis and affect a variety of insects. 0.5 µg of diflubenzuron (DFB; Dimilin) applied topically to female *G. m. morsitans* prevented the production of viable offspring throughout the life of the fly (more than 70 days);

as little as 15 ng within the fly produced abnormal offspring. Such
disruption would seriously affect the population. Tarsal contact is
ineffective (Jordan and Trewern 1978; Jordan *et al*. 1979).

Two analogues of DFB (penfluron and A13-63220) had similar effects.
Larvae produced by treated flies have difficulty pupariating and do
not survive. Radioisotope studies have shown that DFB is stored in
thoracic tissue with low levels in haemolymph, fat body and uterine
gland. Larvae acquire DFB through the uterine milk and the chitin
content of their cuticle is reduced by 70%, almost certainly due to
inhibition of the enzyme chitin synthetase.

The different effects of DFB on *Glossina* depend on the mode of application; aerosol application of 30 µm VMD droplets is optimal. Field
trials are in progress and, if successful, DFB or other IGRs could
provide a new, environmentally acceptable, method of *Glossina* control.
The reduced susceptibility of pregnant female flies to insecticides
suggests that IGRs could be incorporated into the first sequential
application of a series of endosulfan sprays, followed by endosulfan
alone.

8.3.2. Sterile male release method

This method, involving release of large numbers of sterilized male
Glossina bred in the laboratory, depends on the mating competitiveness
of the sterilized males. A small field project using 'wild' pupae and
chemosterilants in Rhodesia (now Zimbabwe) suggested that, with the
development and improvement of mass rearing technology, the release of
large numbers of sterilized males could become a feasible, cost-effective part of an integrated control programme. Since the initial study,
several increasingly large scale projects have been launched; each
had different objectives and, to date, a cost benefit comparison with
other techniques has not been possible. The principles of this method
are described by Knipling (1979); it successfully eradicated screw-
worms (*Cochliomyia hominivorax*) in the south eastern United States.
Sterile male release could possibly be used in *Glossina* control to
'mop-up' the residual elements of a population initially reduced by
sequential non-residual aerosol application (see Van der Vloedt *et al*.
1980 and Dame *et al*. 1980). Eradication, rather than control, should
be the objective, or such projects will not be cost-effective. However, there are problems: really large scale rearing facilities do
not yet exist and the process is labour intensive; the technique is
monospecific and many important vector species or subspecies have not
yet been reared successfully; and rearing depends on a supply of
sterile blood for membrane-feeding of flies or a support colony maintained on goats, guinea pigs or rabbits, the husbandry of which could
be a problem. Logistics of adult and pupal release on a large scale
remain to be assessed - again such requirements are labour intensive
and dependent on reliability of vehicles and increasingly expensive
petrol. Irradiation facilities must be provided. The technique is
not applicable for the control of epidemic human sleeping sickness as
it would take too long to establish a colony; also, it would be

necessary to release fed adult sterile flies, as pupal release might
result in emerged males becoming infected, despite the likelihood of
their reduced longevity; irradiated sterilized and chemosterilized
flies can develop trypanosome infections (Dame and MacKenzie 1968;
Moloo 1982).

Despite advances in rearing techniques (Mews *et al.* 1977), membrane
feeding (Bauer and Wetzel 1976; Wetzel 1979), population sampling
(Challier and Laveissière 1973), and irradiation strategies, such as
irradiation in a nitrogen atmosphere to give increased longevity
(Curtis and Langley 1972), the likelihood of success using this technique even as part of a large scale integrated programme appears
remote. It seems naive to suggest that a technique which has taken
5 years to eradicate a single species of *Glossina* from 40 km of riverine forest (Politzar *et al.* 1979) should be considered promising in
the context of African development programmes, particularly when one
considers the 18 000 km of river where each breeding site of *Simulium*
is treated weekly in the Onchocerciasis Control Programme (Walsh *et*
al. 1979).

Recent sterile male projects have suffered from the problem of
reinvasion from outside the area, despite costly attempts to prevent
this by creating cleared barriers over 1 - 1.3 km. The technique of
spraying the outer perimeter of a barrier with residual insecticide
proved ineffective in Tanzania; flies could cross a 1.3 km linear
barrier in Upper Volta even when traps were placed within them. Reinvasion frequently has prevented a valid assessment of the efficacy
of the technique itself. The difficulty of isolating treated areas
has been highlighted by Curtis (1980); he suggested using the method
to extend progressively an already fly-free area.

8.3.3. Immunization of hosts

Nogge (1976, 1979) immunized rabbits with whole *Glossina m. morsitans*
and tsetse subsequently fed on these rabbits showed increased mortality
and a small decrease in fecundity. However, *Glossina*, and other
haematophagous arthropods, possess symbionts; when rabbits specifically
immunized with these symbionts were used as hosts, the flies showed
much reduced fecundity but no change in longevity. Similarly, Schlein
and Lewis (1976) found an increase in mortality of tsetse fed on
rabbits immunized against various tissues of *Stomoxys*. Interesting
though these results are, it seems unlikely that similar techniques
could be used practically to reduce *Glossina* populations, as every
potential host would need to be immunized.

8.3.4. Traps in control and sampling

Studies in Zimbabwe have identified a component in ox breath which
acts as a powerful olfactory attractant for *G. m. morsitans* and *G.*
pallidipes and clearly demonstrated the potential of traps as control
tools (Vale and Phelps 1978; Hargrove 1980; Vale 1980; Hargrove and
Vale 1980). Vale (1980) has also used acetone and carbon dioxide, in

combination with electrified trapping devices, to enhance the catch
without recourse to ox odour. CO_2 also enhances the catch of biconical
traps (Frezil and Carnevale 1976). None of the ketones or aldehydes
tested was comparable with natural ox breath, and indeed some were
repellent (Vale 1980). The production of a synthetic attractant could
provide a major breakthrough in control. Use of such a chemical in an
odour baited, autosterilizing device using a chemosterilant, with
perhaps the use of the specific female contact sex pheromones recently
described and synthesized (Langley *et al.* 1975; Carlson *et al.* 1978;
Huyton *et al.* 1980), could hold great promise for the future control
of *Glossina*. Such a device could perhaps be developed for *G. palpalis*
group species in West Africa, a sex recognition pheromone having
recently been found in *G. p. palpalis* (Offor *et al.* 1981).

In West and Central Africa emphasis has been on the development and
use of the biconical trap of Challier and Laveissière (1973). Developments in *Glossina* trapping have been reviewed by Challier (1977) and
Hargrove (1977). It has long been known that traps can be used to
control *Glossina*; their use, and handcatching, have been reviewed by
Glasgow and Potts (1970). Ryan *et al.* (1981a) have shown that biconical traps catch approximately 7% of *G. palpalis* and *G. m. centralis*
per day and can contribute to reducing fly populations. The simplicity
and cheapness of the biconical trap has recently reawakened interest
in trapping as a control tool in West Africa, following the earlier
work of Morris (1950) in Ghana using DDT impregnated traps. Laveissière and Couret (1980) found that deltamethrin impregnated biconical
traps could reduce riverine *Glossina* populations by over 99%. Costs
of this technique of control have been estimated at US$ 11 per hectare
in a riverine habitat. This technique might be appropriate for control
in areas of high human sleeping sickness transmission, without recourse
to more sophisticated technology.

Developments in trapping techniques have also provided methods of
estimating relative and absolute efficiency of traps (using electric
grids for capture), and population growth rates (Ryan 1981). Auto-
mation of trapping by incorporating segregating devices and electrified
or insecticide killing units into biconical traps allows fly activity
in relation to traps to be accurately monitored (Ryan *et al.* 1981b).

8.4. Host parasite studies in relation to tsetse and trypanosomiasis

Eradication and/or control of *Glossina* which are transmitting
disease to livestock, though increasingly viewed as a valid economic
venture, can be recommended only in conjunction with rational land
use (Jordan 1979) and the likelihood of a profitable outcome locally
or nationally. It is therefore essential to attempt quantitative
assessment of livestock disease risk, which in the past has been associated with the term 'challenge'. This subject has recently been
reviewed by Rogers (1980) who concluded that there is a linear relationship between apparent density of *Glossina* and incidence of both
human and animal trypanosomiasis.

There is now however evidence that trypanosome infected flies
behave differently from uninfected flies in relation to probing and
feeding frequency (Molyneux *et al*. 1979; Jenni *et al*. 1980). This
has been demonstrated for *T. brucei* by Jenni *et al*. (1980), and Roberts
(1981) has shown that *G. m. morsitans* infected with *T. congolense*
probed more frequently, and took more time to engorge, than uninfected
flies. Infection rates are not an accurate measure of the percentage
of flies which can transmit infection (Harley and Wilson 1968; Otieno
and Darji 1979). It is also known that some species of *Glossina* (*e.g.*
G. brevipalpis), though infected, are very poor transmitters (Wilson
et al. 1972). The fact that a large species of fly such as *G. brevipalpis* is not an efficient transmitter may be due to the food canal
diameter and trypanosome relationships with mechanoreceptors
(Molyneux *et al*. 1979; Jenni *et al*. 1980; Livesey *et al*. 1980); there
may be a direct relationship between diameter of food canal and transmission capability, assuming the parasites are of the same size in
each fly. There is also evidence that *T. brucei* may have an adverse
effect on *Glossina* salivary glands (Golder and Patel 1980), which may
reduce fly longevity. Conversely, there are reports that trypanosome-
infected flies live longer (Baker and Robertson 1957). Maudlin
(1982) has demonstrated that susceptibility to *T. congolense* is an
inherited trait in female *G. m. morsitans*. Possibly the rearing of
fly populations, less susceptible to trypanosome infection, might
contribute to an integrated control approach.

Since Rogers's (1980) review, Ryan *et al*. (1981a) described a method
of estimating absolute population size from an estimate of absolute
trap efficiency, which should provide a more precise estimation of
risk. In addition it is apparent that the behaviour of laboratory-
infected flies differs from that of uninfected flies; other physiological effects of trypanosomes on flies may occur which may alter
earlier assumptions (Golder and Patel 1980; Bursell 1981) on linear
relationships between apparent density and incidence of trypanosomiasis.
Detailed field studies are needed in selected areas to assess all data
relevant to challenge and to provide a precise quantitative approach.

8.5 *Glossina* taxonomy

Highly specific hydrocarbons, identified in the cuticle of tsetse
and other medically important arthropods (Carlson *et al*. 1978; Carlson
and Service 1980; Carlson and Walsh 1981), may provide more refined
tools for identification and taxonomy of *Glossina* than hitherto available. Carlson and Langley (1981) reported that nine species of *Glossina*
could be easily separated, by species and sex, by gas liquid chromato-
graphy of the cuticular paraffins of single flies. Genetic polymorphism is known of some isoenzymes of *Glossina* species and could give
important taxonomic information relevant to epidemiology (Van der
Geest and Kawooya 1975; Gooding 1981).

8.6. Conclusions

This review has attempted to survey areas of the biology of tsetse relevant to disease control. It seems appropriate here to summarize major lacunae and areas where significant progress could be made.

1. The exploitation of olfactory attractants, their synthesis and mass use as an aid to trapping and autosterilizing flies should repay investment; extension of this study to *Glossina palpalis* group flies seems highly desirable.

2. Pilot studies on self-help control using impregnated biconical traps should be initiated, and further studies on the efficiency of traps should be made. Extensive evaluation of cost-effectiveness and community acceptability of traps for human sleeping sickness control should be investigated.

3. There seems little need at the present for new insecticides, although any promising compounds must be tested.

4. There may be a case for the integration of IGRs into control, using fixed wing aircraft in sequential operations; results of field trials are awaited.

5. The danger of developing insecticide resistance should be appreciated, particularly in areas where aerosol techniques result in drift of sublethal doses to downwind *Glossina* populations.

6. Further studies on the genetics of susceptibility of *Glossina* to trypanosomes and comparison of the feeding behaviour of infected and uninfected flies, should lead to more accurate assessment of risk. This would help in judging the advisability of developing particular areas, and the economic benefit which might accrue from control measures in such areas.

7. Despite the limited success of sterile male programmes, assessment of the value of the technique is difficult as economic data are not yet available. The larger scale programmes now in progress should provide these, and indicate the logistic feasibility of such an approach in areas where more than one species occurs and where re-invasion cannot be reduced by artificial barriers.

8. Recent environmental studies have indicated the side effects of those pesticides in common use, the indicator species to be studied are known and methods to mitigate the side effects of pesticides have been defined.

9. Biological control through parasitoids or predators is not of great potential value in the near future, in view of the promising developments in other areas (*e.g.* traps).

However, the difficulties remain of transferring laboratory results to the field, and applying satisfactorily those measures which are known to be effective. The inadequacies which exist, therefore, usually result from the failure of Governments to recognise the problem as one in which funds should be invested; if, as in countries such as Nigeria and Zimbabwe, there has been such recognition, the economic advantage of effective measures is evident. Many Governments, however, require funds for training personnel; for if programmes based on available technology are to be developed, appropriately trained manpower and the facility to maintain that manpower at the necessary level of motivation and skill, are required. Finally, it must be recognised that tsetse control is only one component of any rural development programme; the responsibilities of planners in this regard should be emphasized at an early stage. The overall objective should be to use the best technique available now; and, if a technique becomes available that is more cost-effective, to integrate it, after suitable trial, into control or eradication.

Acknowledgements

I am grateful to Drs A.M. Jordan, S.L. Croft and L. Ryan for comments on the manuscript.

8.7. References

Baker, J.R. and Robertson, D.H.H. (1957). An experiment on the infectivity to *Glossina morsitans* of a strain of *Trypanosoma rhodesiense* and of a strain of *Trypanosoma brucei* with some observations on the longevity of infected flies. Annals of Tropical Medicine and Parasitology 51, 121-125.

Baldry, D.A.T., Molyneux, D.H. and Van Wettere, P. (1978). The experimental application of insecticides from a helicopter for the control of riverine populations of *Glossina tachinoides* in West Africa. V. Evaluation of decamethrin applied as a spray. Pesticides Abstracts and News Summary 24, 447-454.

Baldry, D.A.T., Everts, J., Roman, B., Boon von Ochsee, G.A. and Laveissière, C. (1981). The experimental application of insecticides from a helicopter for the control of riverine populations of *Glossina tachinoides* in West Africa. Part VIII: The effects of two spray applications of OMS-570 (endosulfan) and of OMS-1998 (decamethrin) on *G. tachinoides* and non-target organisms in Upper Volta. Tropical Pest Management 27, 83-110.

Bauer, B. and Wetzel, H. (1976). A new membrane for feeding *Glossina morsitans* Westw. (Diptera: Glossinidae). Bulletin of Entomological Research 65, 563-565.

Bursell, E. (1981). Energetics of haematophagous arthropods: influence of parasites. Parasitology 82, 107-108.

Carlson, D.A. and Langley, P.A. (1981). Chemical taxonomy in *Glossina* species. Presented at International Scientific Committee for Trypanosomiasis Research and Control, October 1981, Arusha, Tanzania.

Carlson, D.A. and Service, M.W. (1980). Identification of mosquitoes of *Anopheles gambiae* species complex A and B by analysis of cuticular components. Science 207, 1089-1091.

Carlson, D.A. and Walsh, J.F. (1981). Identification of two West African black flies (Diptera: Simuliidae) of the *Simulium damnosum* species complex by analysis of cuticular hydrocarbons. Acta Tropica 38, 235-239.

Carlson, D.A., Langley, P.A. and Huyton, P. (1978). Sex pheromone of the tsetse fly: isolation, identification, and synthesis of contact aphrodisiacs. Science 201, 750-753.

Challier, A. (1965). Amélioration de la méthode de détermination de l'age physiologique des glossines. Études faites sur *Glossina palpalis gambiensis* (Vanderplank, 1949). Bulletin de la Société de Pathologie Exotique 58, 250-259.

Challier, A. (1977). Trapping technology, in Tsetse: The Future for Biological Methods in Integrated Control (edited by M. Laird), pp. 109-123. International Development Research Centre, Ottawa (Publication no. IDRC-D77e).

Challier, A. and Laveissière, C. (1973). Un nouveau piège pour la capture de glossines (*Glossina*: Diptera, Muscidae): déscription et essais sur le terrain. Cahiers ORSTOM Séries Entomologie Médicale et Parasitologie 11, 251-262.

Chapin, G. and Wasserstrom, R. (1981). Agricultural production and malaria resurgence in Central America and India. Nature 293, 181-185.

Curtis, C.F. (1980). Factors affecting the efficiency of the sterile male release method for tsetse, in Isotope and Radiation Research on Animal Diseases and their Vectors. Proceedings of a Symposium No. 240, pp. 381-396. International Atomic Energy Agency, Vienna.

Curtis, C.F. and Langley, P.A. (1972). Use of nitrogen and chilling in the production of radiation-induced sterility in the tsetse fly *Glossina morsitans*. Entomologica Experimentalis et Applicata 15, 360-376.

Dame, D.A. and MacKenzie, P.K.I. (1968). Transmission of *Trypanosoma congolense* by chemosterilised male *G. morsitans*. Annals of Tropical Medicine and Parasitology 62, 372-376.

Dame, D.A., Williamson, D.L., Cobb, P.C., Gates, D.B., Warner, P.B., Mtuya, A.S. and Baumgartner, H. (1980). Integration of sterile insects and pesticides for the control of the tsetse fly *Glossina morsitans morsitans*, in Isotopes and Radiation Research on Animal Diseases and their Vectors. Proceedings of a Symposium No. 240, pp. 267-280. International Atomic Energy Agency, Vienna.

Davies, H. (1964). Eradication of tsetse in the Chad River system of Northern Nigeria. Journal of Applied Ecology 1, 387-403.

Davies, H. (1971). Further eradication of tsetse in the Chad and Gongola River Systems in north-eastern Nigeria. Journal of Applied Ecology 8, 573-578.

98

Davies, J.E. (1978). The use of ageing techniques to evaluate the effects of aerial spraying against *Glossina morsitans centralis* Machado (Diptera: Glossinidae) in Northern Botswana. Bulletin of Entomological Research 68, 373-384.

Davies, J.E. (1981). Insecticide drift and reinvasion of spray blocks in aerial spray experiments against *Glossina morsitans centralis* Machado (Diptera: Glossinidae). Bulletin of Entomological Research 71, 499-508.

Du Toit, R. (1954). Trypanosomiasis in Zululand and control of tsetse flies by chemical means. Onderstepoort Journal of Veterinary Research 26, 317-387.

Elliott, M., Jones, N.F. and Potter, C. (1978). The future of pyrethroids in insect control. Annual Review of Entomology 23, 443-469.

FAO (1977). Insecticide and Application Equipment for Tsetse Control (FAO Animal Production and Health Paper 3). Food and Agriculture Organization of the United Nations, Rome.

FAO (1981). Report of the Panel of Experts on Development Aspects of the Programme for the Control of African Animal Trypanosomiasis and Related Development. Food and Agriculture Organization of the United Nations, Rome.

Frézil, J.L. and Carnevale, P. (1976). Utilisation de la carboglace pour la capture de *Glossina fuscipes quanzensis* Rives 1948 avec la piège Challier-Laveissière: conséquences épidémiologique. Cahiers ORSTOM Séries Entomologie Médicale et Parasitologie 14, 225-233.

Ford, J. (1971). The Role of the Trypanosomiases in African Ecology. Clarendon Press, Oxford.

Glasgow, J.P. and Potts, W.H. (1970). Control by handcatching and traps, in The African Trypanosomiases (edited by H.W. Mulligan), pp. 456-463. George Allen and Unwin, London.

Golder, T. and Patel, N. (1980). Some effects of trypanosome development in the saliva and salivary glands of the tsetse fly *G. morsitans*. European Journal of Cell Biology 22, 511.

Gooding, R.H. (1981). Genetic polymorphism in three species of tsetse flies (Diptera: Glossinidae) in Upper Volta. Acta Tropica 38, 149-161.

Hargrove, J.W. (1977). Some advances in the trapping of tsetse (*Glossina* spp.) and other flies. Ecological Entomology 2, 123-127.

Hargrove, J.W. (1980). The effect of model size and ox odour on the alighting response of *Glossina morsitans* Westwood and *G. pallidipes* Austen (Diptera: Glossinidae). Bulletin of Entomological Research 70, 229-234.

Hargrove, J.W. and Vale, G.A. (1980). Catches of *Glossina morsitans morsitans* Westwood and *G. pallidipes* Austen (Diptera: Glossinidae) in odour-baited traps in riverine and deciduous woodlands in the Zambesi Valley of Zimbabwe. Bulletin of Entomological Research 70, 571-578.

Harley, J.M.B. and Wilson, A.J. (1968). Comparison between *Glossina morsitans*, *G. pallidipes* and *G. fuscipes* as vectors of trypanosomes of the *Trypanosoma congolense* group: the proportions infected experimentally and the numbers of infective organisms extruded during feeding. Annals of Tropical Medicine and Parasitology 62, 178-187.

Huyton, P.M., Langley, P.A., Carlson, D.A. and Scharz, M. (1980). Specificity of contact sex pheromone in tsetse flies *Glossina* spp. Physiological Entomology 5, 253-264.

Jenni, L., Molyneux, D.H., Livesey, J.L. and Galun, R. (1980). Feeding behaviour of tsetse flies infected with salivarian trypanosomes. Nature 283, 383-385.

Jordan, A.M. (1974). Recent developments in the ecology and methods of control of tsetse flies (*Glossina* spp.) (Dipt., Glossinidae) - a review. Bulletin of Entomological Research 63, 361-399.

Jordan, A.M. (1976). Tsetse flies as vectors of trypanosomes. Veterinary Parasitology 2, 143-152.

Jordan, A.M. (1978). Principles of the eradication or control of tsetse flies. Nature 273, 607-609.

Jordan, A.M. (1979). Trypanosomiasis control and land use in Africa. Outlook on Agriculture 10, 123-129.

Jordan, A.M. and Trewern, M.A. (1978). Larvicidal activity of diflubenzuron in the tsetse fly, *Glossina morsitans morsitans* Westw. Nature 245, 462.

Jordan, A.M., Trewern, M.A., Borkovec, A.B. and DeMilo, A.B. (1979). Laboratory studies on the potential of three insect growth regulators for control of the tsetse fly, *Glossina morsitans morsitans* Westwood (Diptera: Glossinidae). Bulletin of Entomological Research 69, 55-64.

Knipling, E.F. (1979). The Basic Principles of Insect Population Suppression and Management (Agricultural Handbook No. 512). United States Department of Agriculture, Washington, D.C.

Koeman, J.H., Balk, F. and Takken, W. (1980). The Environmental Impact of Tsetse Control Operations. A Report on Present Knowledge (FAO Animal Production and Health Paper 7, first revision). Food and Agriculture Organization of the United Nations, Rome.

Laird, M., editor (1977). Tsetse: The Future for Biological Methods in Integrated Control. International Development Research Centre, Ottawa (Publication no. IDRC-077e).

Langley, P.A., Pimley, R.W. and Carlson, D.A. (1975). Sex recognition pheromone in tsetse fly *Glossina morsitans*. Nature 254, 51-53.

Laveissière, C. and Couret, D. (1980). Traps impregnated with insecticide for the control of riverine tsetse flies. Transactions of the Royal Society of Tropical Medicine and Hygiene 74, 264-265.

100

Lee, C. (1977). New developments in tsetse fly control using aircraft. Agricultural Aviation 18, 6-17.

Lee, C.W., Parker, J.D., Baldry, D.A.T. and Molyneux, D.H. (1978). The experimental application of insecticides from a helicopter for the control of riverine populations of *Glossina tachinoides* in West Africa. II. Calibration of equipment and insecticide dispersal. Pesticides Abstracts and News Summary 24, 404-422.

Lee, C.W., Parker, J.D., Kutzer, H., Baldry, D.A.T., Bettany, B.W. and Tunstall, J. (1980). The experimental application of insecticides from a helicopter for the control of riverine populations of *Glossina tachinoides* in West Africa. VII. Studies on the physical properties of sprays of Endosulfan and Deltamethrin applied to *G. tachinoides* habitats in the R. Komoe Valley, Upper Volta. Tropical Pest Management 26, 377-384.

Livesey, J.L., Molyneux, D.H. and Jenni, L. (1980). Mechanoreceptor-trypanosome interactions in the labrum of *Glossina*: fluid mechanics. Acta Tropica 37, 151-161.

MacLennan, K.J.R. (1981). Tsetse transmitted trypanosomiasis in relation to the rural economy in Africa. II. Techniques in use for the control or eradication of tsetse infestations. World Animal Review 37, 9-91.

Mattheissen, P. (1981). Haematological changes in fish following aerial spraying with endosulfan insecticide for tsetse fly control in Botswana. Journal of Fish Biology 18, 461-469.

Maudlin, I. (1982). Inheritance of susceptibility to *Trypanosoma congolense* infection in *Glossina morsitans*. Annals of Tropical Medicine and Parasitology 76, 225-228.

Maudlin, I., Green, C. and Barlow, F. (1981). The potential for insecticide resistance in *Glossina* (Diptera: Glossinidae) - an investigation by computer simulation and chemical analysis. Bulletin of Entomological Research 71, 691-702.

Mews, A.R., Langley, P.A., Pimley, R.W. and Flood, M.E.T. (1977). Large-scale rearing of tsetse flies (*Glossina* spp.) in the absence of a living host. Bulletin of Entomological Research 67, 119-128.

Moloo, S.K. (1982). Cyclical transmission of pathogenic *Trypanosoma* species by gamma-irradiated sterile male *Glossina morsitans morsitans* Parasitology 84, 289-296.

Molyneux, D.H. (1977). Vector relationships in the Trypanosomatidae. Advances in Parasitology 15, 1-82.

Molyneux, D.H., Baldry, D.A.T., De Raadt, P., Lee, C.W. and Hamon, J. (1978). Helicopter application of insecticides for the control of riverine *Glossina* vectors of African human trypanosomiasis in the moist savannah zones. Annales de la Société Belge de Médecine Tropicale 58, 185-203.

Molyneux, D.H., Lavin, D.R. and Elce, B. (1979). A possible relation-ship between salivarian trypanosomes and *Glossina* labrum mechano-receptors. Annals of Tropical Medicine and Parasitology 73, 287-290.

Morris, M.G. (1950). The persistance of toxicity on DDT impregnated hessian and its use on tsetse traps. Bulletin of Entomological Research 41, 259-288.

Moss, R.P. and Morgan, W.B. (1981). Fuelwood and rural energy prod-uction and supply in the humid tropics. Natural Resources and the Environment Series, volume 4. Tycooly International Publishing, Dublin (for the United Nations University).

Mulligan, H.W., editor (1970). The African Trypanosomiases. George Allen and Unwin, London.

Nogge, G. (1976). Sterility in tsetse flies (*Glossina morsitans* Westwood) caused by loss of symbionts. Experientia 32, 995.

Nogge, G. (1978). Aposymbiotic tsetse flies, *Glossina morsitans morsitans* obtained by feeding on rabbits immunized specifically with symbionts. Journal of Insect Physiology 24, 299-304.

Offor, I.I., Carlson, D.A., Gadzama, N.M. and Bozimo, H.T. (1981). Sex recognition pheromone in the West African tsetse fly *Glossina palpalis palpalis* (Robineau-Desvoïdy). Insect Science and its Application 1, 417-420.

Otieno, L.H. (1978). The presence in salivary secretions of *Glossina morsitans* of stages of *Trypanosoma (Trypanozoon) brucei* other than those occurring in the salivary glands. Transactions of the Royal Society of Tropical Medicine and Hygiene 72, 622-626.

Otieno, L.H. and Darji, N. (1979). The abundance of pathogenic African trypanosomes in the salivary secretions of wild *Glossina pallidipes*. Annals of Tropical Medicine and Parasitology 73, 583-588.

Politzar, H., Cuisance, D., Lafaye, A., Clair, M., Taze, Y. and Sellin, E. (1979). Expérimentation sur le terrain de la lutte génétique par lâchers de mâles stériles: longevité et dispersion des mâles irradiés de *Glossina palpalis gambiensis* (Haute-Volta). Annales de la Société Belge de Médecine Tropicale 59, 59-78.

Quinlan, R.J. and Gatehouse, A.G. (1981a). Characteristics and implications of knockdown of the tsetse fly *Glossina morsitans morsitans* Westw. by Deltamethrin. Pesticide Science 12, 439-442.

Quinlan, R.J. and Gatehouse, A.G. (1981b). The effect of low doses of Endosulfan on lipid reserves of the tsetse fly *Glossina morsitans morsitans*. Entomologia Experimentalis et Applicata 29, 29-38.

Roberts, L.W. (1981). Probing by *Glossina morsitans morsitans* and transmission of *Trypanosoma (Nannomonas) congolense*. American Journal of Tropical Medicine and Hygiene 30, 948-951.

Roche, L. (1975). Forestry and the conservation of plants and animals in the tropics. Forest Ecology and Management 2, 103-122.

Rogers, D.J. (1980). Trypanosomiasis 'risk' or 'challenge'. A review with recommendations. AGA:TRYP/80/Rep.4. Food and Agriculture Organization of the United Nations, Rome. [Mimeographed.]

Russell-Smith, A. and Ruckert, E. (1981). The effects of aerial spraying of endosulfan for tsetse fly control on aquatic invertebrates in the Okavango swamps, Botswana. Environmental Pollution, Series A 24, 57-73.

Ryan, L. (1981). *Glossina* (Diptera: Glossinidae) population growth rates. Bulletin of Entomological Research 71, 519-531.

Ryan, L., Molyneux, D.H., Kuzoe, F.A.S. and Baldry, D.A.T. (1981a). Traps to control and estimate populations of *Glossina*. Tropenmedizin und Parasitologie 32, 145-148.

Ryan, L., Molyneux, D.H., Harrison, N. and Hillier, M. (1981b). An automatic tsetse (Diptera: Glossinidae) trap. Tropical Pest Management 27, 111-115.

Schlein, Y. and Lewis, C.T. (1979). Lesions in haematophagous flies after feeding on rabbits immunised with fly tissues. Physiological Entomology 1, 55-59.

Spielberger, U., Na'Isa, B.K., Koch, K. and Manno, A. (1979). Field trials with the synthetic pyrethroids permethrin, cypermethrin and decamethrin against *Glossina* (Diptera: Glossinidae) in Nigeria. Bulletin of Entomological Research 69, 667-689.

Vale, G.A. (1980). Field studies of the responses of tsetse flies (Glossinidae) and other Diptera to carbon dioxide, acetone and other chemicals. Bulletin of Entomological Research 70, 563-570.

Vale, G.A. and Phelps, R.J. (1978). Sampling problems with tsetse flies. Journal of Applied Ecology 15, 715-726.

Van der Geest, L.P.S. and Kawooya, J. (1975). Genetic variation in some enzyme systems in the tsetse fly *Glossina morsitans*. Entomologia Experimentalis et Applicata 18, 508-514.

Van der Vloedt, A.M.V., Baldry, D.A.T., Politzar, H., Kulzer, H. and Cuisance, D. (1980). Experimental helicopter applications of decamethrin followed by release of sterile males for the control of riverine vectors of trypanosomiasis in Upper Volta. Insect Science and its Application 1, 105-112.

Van Wettere, P., Baldry, D.A.T., Moylneux, D.H., Clarke, J.H., Lee, C.W. and Parker, J.D. (1978). The experimental application of insecticides from a helicopter for the control of riverine populations of *Glossina tachinoides* in West Africa. IV. Evaluation of insecticides applied as aerosols. Pesticides Abstracts and News Summary 24, 435-446.

Walsh, J.F., Davies, J.B. and Le Berre, R. (1979). Entomological aspects of the first five years of the Onchocerciasis Control Programme in the Volta River Basin. Tropenmedizin und Parasitologie 30, 328-344.

Wetzel, H. (1979). Artificial membrane for *in vitro* feeding of piercing-sucking arthropods. Entomologia Experimentalis et Applicata 25, 117-119

Index